@PaulRuebig ■ @AchimKaspar

EMERGENCY PREPAREDNESS

A Sustainable #Food #WATER #Energy Future

TRAUNER

IMPRINT

All information is provided without a warranty. The authors are responsible for the accuracy and completeness of the content. Any liability of the authors, the editors, and the publisher is not included.

© 2023
by KR Dr. Paul Rübig fMEP, Wels

All image rights, unless otherwise stated, are held by the editor.

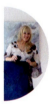

Cover image:
"The Wave" von Ulli Perner,
Kunst zwischen den Seen,
Dimension: 100 x 80 cm,
www.ulli-perner.at

Publishing house and distribution:
TRAUNER Verlag + Buchservice GmbH
Köglstraße 14, 4020 Linz
Österreich/Austria

Production:
Druckerei Salzkammergut-Media Ges.m.b.H.
Druckereistraße 4, 4810 Gmunden

PRINTED IN
AUSTRIA

ISBN 978-3-99113-867-9
www.trauner.at

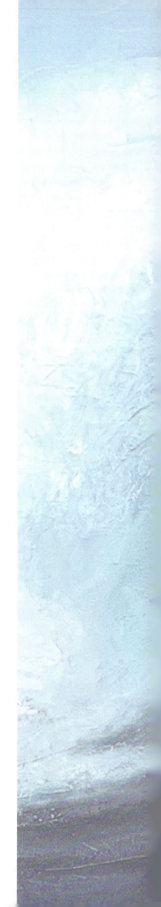

@PaulRuebig ▪ @AchimKaspar

EMERGENCY PREPAREDNESS

A Sustainable #Food #WATER #Energy Future

ACKNOWLEDGEMENTS

We are grateful to **DI Bruno Lindorfer**, former Chief Research Officer of Siemens VAI Metals Technologies and CEO of the Upper Austrian Innovation and Technology GmbH for his expertise and continuous support throughout the creation of the four EESC Opinions, without which this book would have not come to life.

We extend our utmost gratitude to **Sabine Seidel, MA**, for her outstanding contribution to this book. Sabine's project and author coordination, project management, and tireless efforts were instrumental in bringing this project to fruition. Her dedication, expertise, and attention to detail helped ensure the success of this joint work. Sabine's ability to manage complex logistics and coordinate diverse stakeholders was truly indispensable. Your contribution has made a lasting impact, and we are honored to have had the opportunity to have you onboard this project.

Our sincere appreciation shall also be expressed to **Dr. Horst Heitz**, Executive Director of the SME Europe of the EPP, for his active participation in the developmental process of this compilation. His extensive professional network, expertise in the field and countless vital suggestions throughout the drafting process were invaluable to the project.

THE EDITORS

▌ KR Ing. Mag. Dr. Paul Rübig, fMEP

born in Wels (Upper Austria), entrepreneur and educated as an agricultural engineer in the HTL Steyr, Business Administration JKU Linz, Dean WIFI OÖ (dual education), regional Assembly, national Parliament, member of the European Parliament from 1996 to 2019. He is married and has two children.

In the European Parliament, Paul Rübig was a full member of the Committee on Industry, Research and Energy, and the Committee on Budgets. In addition, he was a substitute member of the Committee on Development and the Committee on International Trade and Co-Chair of the Steering Group of the Parliamentary Conference on the WTO. He was Chairman of STOA (Scientific Technology Options Assessment) – Panel for the Future of Science and Technology, an official body of the European Parliament that is supported by external experts such as universities, scientists, or research institutes. Three time winner of the "MEP of the Year"-Award in 2008, 2013, and 2015, organised by the Parliament Magazine, DodsGroup.

Paul Rübig is very active in the field of small-scale business promotion. He is president of SME Global, a working group of the International Democrat Union (IDU), whose objective it is to support small and medium-sized enterprises (SME) and to improve their business environments.

In 2019 Paul Rübig was appointed to the Advisory Board of Rübig Holding GmbH and he enjoys SDG6 related investments.

In 2022 Paul Rübig was appointed as External Advisor to the Board of Directors of Water Europe and is a member of IWA.

Member of the Governing Board of the European Institute of Innovation and Technology, Budapest.

A new KIC, in the field of Water, Marine, and Maritime Sectors and Ecosystems, is proposed to be launched in 2026, with a call for proposals to be published in 2025.

Member of the European Economic and Social Committee, Brussels.

As member of the Conference on the Future of Europe he supported an EU Competitiveness Test.

▌ Dr. Achim Kaspar

is Member of the Board of VERBUND AG – Austria's leading electricity company and one of the largest producers of electricity from hydropower in Europe. He assumed the role as COO in January 2019 and is responsible for digitisation as well as the VERBUND generation portfolio which includes the oversight of 130 hydropower plants.

Prior to joining VERBUND, he held various management positions in the Utility and Service Provider Industry as well as in the Austrian Telecommunication Industry.

From 2008–2018 Achim Kaspar was General Manager at Cisco Austria / Slovenia / Croatia.

∎ 7 AFFORDABLE AND CLEAN ENERGY

∎ 14 LIFE BELOW WATER

TECHNOLOGY, ENGINEERING AND EDUCATION

#EMERGENCYPREPAREDNESS #ERA #INNOVATION #RESEARCH #5MISSIONS

The world is changing every day, and we must find good options for our future. **Options Assessment** with the right **Foresight Strategy** could help to make the right decisions. With **Impact Assessment** studies we can learn how to do better and use **Risk Assessment** for the best solutions. The sustainable development goals need a lot of innovation to have a good return of investment and the people's income. We need food and feed, water and sanitation, wastewater mining, renewable and efficient energy production, and a clean and blue economy ocean.

The European Research Area, the research and innovation strategy together with the five missions, can help to increase awareness of **Emergency Preparedness** and new technologies with higher education, skills, and vocational training. The value chain and **Lifetime Cycles Studies** should promote a global development of sustainability with a SME and **competitiveness Test**. From university to kindergarten, we have to use the existing knowledge in combination with new learning and teaching technologies.

SMEs and Family Business can play a big role in the development of individual, personalised solutions with services and products which could be chosen by informed consumers. Therefore, we decided to produce a knowledge-driven book with scientists, researchers, and innovative entrepreneurs to help to understand what taxpayers should finance and how citizens can benefit. All institutions and organisations are responsible for delivering the right answers.

Just do it. Let's start a new process with financial engineering, databases, and machine learning to predict a trusted future.

Paul Rübig
(Editor)

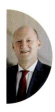

THERE IS NO LIFE WITHOUT WATER

A simple chemical compound is the major component of our lives. H_2O is omnipresent in all states of aggregation, solid as well as liquid and gaseous. You can see it, grab it, feel it – and water is able to taste fantastic, too.

The benefits of water resources are manifold. We can use or consume water, but we are also able to contaminate water or to wastewater. Today the only valid position can be a careful and sustainable use of water and a great respect for our water resources. Everybody can and has to contribute. First, everone can optimise their own consumption, and second, they can try to raise awareness and shape opinions for different usage, tasks, and problems in their surrounding or specific field. By presenting a wealth of information about the diverse applications and interconnectedness of water, this book aims to empower readers to take action and make a positive impact on water resources.

You will get useful insights and exciting information about the actual status quo and the next possible and/or necessary steps for sustainable development. Every chapter is a valuable source and all authors deliver an important input for the necessary creation of political awareness and elucidation. After you have read this book, you will have further knowledge in water-related topics such as biodiversity, water security challenges and solutions, and water management. You will also have knowledge about using the energy of hydropower, which is at the core of our sustainable technologies.

Worldwide electricity generation in 2020 measured approx. 26.800 TWh, but only about 28 % of the amount was produced from regenerative resources. In detail, the major part – 58 % – of the worldwide renewable electricity production was produced by hydropower, with an output of 4.347 TWh. Hydropower plants have the highest advantages, qualities, and power spectrum within the renewable family, e.g. sustainability, security of supply, flexibility, system stability. Hydropower generation is also a very important factor to help reach the sustainable development goals of SDG 7 clean energy, SDG 12 responsible production, and SDG 13 climate action by compensating fossil fuels.

H_2O is directly and indirectly the lifeblood for all plants, animals, and humans. It is an integral part of every life and the engine for our climate. Water is our most important and valuable resource. So let´s ensure a sustainable development. Today we have to choose the right paths for the next generation. That means that we have to make appropriate steps to keep the Earth and all of its lifeforms alive.

Achim Kaspar
(Editor)

DEAR READERS,

As President of the European Economic and Social Committee (EESC), I would like to congratulate Paul Rübig. His very timely book, once more, proves his foresight in economic and societal challenges at regional, national, and European levels.

Access to water has been something we have taken for granted in major parts of Europe. In recent years, with the consequences of climate change becoming more apparent, water has become an increasingly political topic of discussion given its impact not only on the planet but also on our economies and societies. Water has become an increasingly scarce resource. Access to water, water quality, water use, and water consumption needs to be given the corresponding political attention.

More than a billion people worldwide still do not have access to drinking water. 80 % of wastewater is discharged untreated into the environment, and more than 90 % of natural disasters are water related. In Europe, 7 people die daily from diarrheal diseases due to unsafe or inadequate drinking water, sanitation, and hygiene. The gap between global water supply and demand is projected to reach 40 % by 2030, if current practices continue.

Natural disasters were prevalent throughout the summer of 2022, when droughts, forest fires, and floods were reported all over Europe. We are currently living in challenging times, with climate change, war in Europe, and the Covid pandemic. The availability and sustainable management of water impacts global health, migration, social peace, and societal as well as economic progress and business.

Water conservation will require a real change in how we live, how agriculture and businesses across sectors use water, and how we set our policies. The EESC has worked on various issues surrounding water, while always keeping the interest of organised civil society at the forefront. The United Nations 2023 Water Conference will take place next year. Goal 6 of the Sustainable Development Goals is to ensure the availability and sustainable management of water. If Europe wants to be a frontrunner of climate change, we have to make this goal a reality!

I wish you an insightful and interesting read.

Christa Schweng
(EESC President)

A BRIEF POLICY COMMENT ON THE GLOBAL IMPORTANCE OF WATER MANAGEMENT

Water is the most precious and essential natural resource. If there is no water, there would be no life on Earth. Like any resource, water can become scarce, especially when demand for water exceeds supply or poor quality limits its use. This particularly affects the valuable fresh water, since only 0.3 percent on Earth is usable for humans.

Innovative and sustainable water management is now more important than ever. Environmental protection as well as climate protection and migration policy are global issues. Thus, water management is becoming a global instrument. Safe and readily available water is important for public health, whether it is used for drinking, domestic use, food production, or recreational purposes. Large supplies of water are needed by industries for fabricating, processing, washing, diluting, cooling, or transporting a product. All topics also have a high potential for conflict and are directly or at least indirectly linked to migration and security policy. Whether in Jordan, in the future of the Nile water, in the Euphrates and Tigris, in the Andes, in the Himalayas between China and India, in Africa, or in regard to climate change – the list can go on eternally. In this context is no surprise that there is always a chapter on water in almost every international strategy or agreement.

This short text shows how complex, diverse, and fundamental the topic of water is for us humans. But what does this mean in concrete terms for water management and politics?

Firstly, let's take a look at Europe, which also faces challenges when it comes to water. Around 80 % of Europe's freshwater (both drinking and other) comes from rivers and groundwater, which can also make these sources vulnerable to threats from overexploitation, pollution, and climate change. In some regions of Europe, there has long been a need for investment in their water management and technology. A new extreme case is Ukraine. Due to the Russian attack on this country and the terror against its civil infrastructure, additional investments in the billions are now necessary for reconstruction there alone. Despite all the tragedy, this also offers an opportunity to modernise Ukrainian water management, especially for industrial water and agriculture.

Let us now turn to Africa. The EU wants to move away from classic development policy towards strategic partnerships with associated large-scale investments. The financing of nationwide infrastructure should lead to state stability and economic prosperity – in this way, causes of flight should also be avoided. Investing in the water management of this continent is of fundamental interest to Europe. The African continent is ecologically very diverse. Climate change will further increase the pressure on water resources, affect biodiversity and human health, worsen food security, and increase desertification. Adaptation to climate change is therefore an urgent necessity for Africa's development. But also in the global fight against pandemics and resistant germs, African regions with weak infrastructure will inevitably come into the focus of the world community and thus also the water industry.

Another part of the world of greatest European interest is the Middle East and North Africa (MENA). This region is the driest area on Earth and has already been affected by desertification, overexploitation of groundwater, and seawater intrusion into aquifers. In addition, the consequences of climate change for the water supply in the MENA region will intensify, and the expected population and economic growth by 2035 will probably lead to an increase in water demand by 47 %. In the MENA region, agriculture accounts for more than 80 % of freshwater consumption. Water conflicts could therefore massively threaten stability there and thus also have direct consequences for Europe.

To complete the global view, let's take a quick look at South America and Asia. The Regulatory Authority estimates that Brazil alone would have to invest at least 4 billion US dollars per year in its water management. Things are no better in neighbouring Argentina, not to mention Uruguay, Bolivia, and Mexico. China and India also have an immense amount of catching up to do and require huge investments – be it in the drinking water supply, sewage management, or irrigation. The situation is no different in most other Asian countries (with a few exceptions).

These global challenges require research, innovation, and entrepreneurship at the highest level. However, this also offers enormous future opportunities for small and medium-sized companies from this sector, especially from Europe. Our SMEs have enormous potential and demonstrate their know-how in a wide variety of projects worldwide. At the same time, this is a task for European politics to continue to maintain and create the best framework conditions in the EU for these entrepreneurs – not only for the European internal market but also with regard to being able to successfully face international competition. The success of the latter also means that these entrepreneurs engage in international and regional networks in order to become part of the increasingly institutionalised global water community and its project landscape. The exchange of knowledge, experience, and contacts should form the basis of such cooperation and is therefore a very important prerequisite for SMEs to be successful in the various regions of the world.

The approach to networking, as in the case of the SME Connect SDG6 group, has a model character for me. At this point, I would therefore like to expressly thank Dr. Paul Rübig for his initiative and commitment to building this SME group. I wish you continued success and will continue to support this project.

Ivan Štefanec
(President SME Europe)

"WATER IS LIFE"

"Water is life" is a sentence we have all heard countless times. Everybody nods in agreement when people discuss the value of water. How though can we separate how valuable we consider water for our lives from our actions to protect it? Availability, quality, and accessibility of water are still too often taken for granted the moment that water is just a limited resource.

Today, floods, droughts, water pollution, and water scarcity make it to the news as the everyday challenges that our planet faces. But these problems are a lot bigger than just headlines. We need solutions to address the rising challenges. We need investments and technological and non-technological innovations. Still, most importantly, we need a combination of all of these. This book is being published at a time when we need to go one step beyond the discussions, the questions, and the whys and dive into the answers to our challenges. The pages that you will go through do exactly that by offering a detailed compilation of the solutions and best practices from experts in the water management field.

No matter whether our well-being, the economy, the environment, or food security is the topic, water is the foundation from which everything starts. "Follow the water" has been one of the guiding principles in the search for extraterrestrial life, so how can we ignore it on our own blue planet?

Durk Krol
(Executive Managing Director of Water Europe)

EMERGENCY MANAGEMENT

At the European Parliamentary Research Service (EPRS), the Think Tank of the European Parliament, I had the pleasure of pioneering foresight. At EPRS, we could do so with and due to the enthusiastic support of the political side of the European Parliament, especially from Dr. Paul Rübig, who was the Chair of European Parliament's Science and Technology Options Assessment (STOA) Panel. He became a persuasive foresight ambassador.

In today's fast changing world, we see more and more that science has its limitations. Not all technological developments, however promising, are unconditionally welcomed by everyone. Not all of them are good for society overall; not all of them are good for individual human beings. Therefore, responsible policymaking should not only be directed by science. It has to consider the possible impact of new developments on society. Foresight methods allow us to balance scientific evidence with the societal context. And I am glad that foresight-based methods for policy analysis have been gaining attention in European institutions. With a growing awareness for citizens' hopes and fears, we have moved from evidence-based policymaking to foresight-based policymaking, which—in my view—makes policy more human.

Dr. Rübig applies such foresight methods to his daily work at the European Economic and Social Committee and to his activities on emergency preparedness, while addressing the United Nation's Sustainable Development Goals. He focuses on emergencies—such as water shortages, power outages, and cyberthreats—using a foresight-based approach, while considering the possible impact of the events on a wide range of actors and mapping the vulnerabilities of the different players within the society. He develops proposals for handling the entire range of phases of emergency management—namely prevention, preparedness, response, mitigation, and recovery—on different time horizons in order to tackle crises.

Water resilience, the main topic of Dr. Rübig's book, is the most important issue of emergency preparation, which has also been highlighted as a major global risk in the European Parliament's "Future Shocks 2023" report.

This book will be a valuable read for policymakers dealing with emergency management.

Lieve Van Woensel
(Former Foresight Advisor, European Parliamentary Research Service)

EUROPEAN ECONOMIC AND SOCIAL COMMITTEE OPINIONS

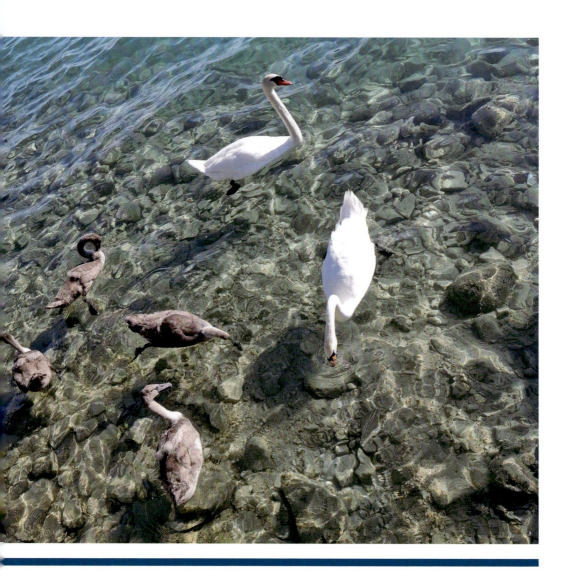

INT/989

OPINION EUROPEAN ECONOMIC AND SOCIAL COMMITTEE
EMERGENCY PREPAREDNESS

Paul Rübig

Members: Pietro Vittorio Barbieri (IT-Gr. III) (Rule 86(2) – Rodert), Giulia Barbucci (IT-Gr. II) (Rule 86(2) – Mone), Dimitris Dimitriadis (EL-Gr. I), Panagiotis Gkofas (EL-Gr. III), Thomas Kattnig (AT-Gr. II) (Rule 86(2) – Reisecker), Thierry Libaert (FR-Gr. III), Aurel Laurenţiu Plosceanu (RO-Gr. I) (Rule 86(2) – Muresan), Christophe Quarez (FR-Gr. II) (Rule 86(2) – Meynent), Wautier Robyns de Schneiderauer (BE-Gr. I), Ferre Wyckmans (BE-Gr. II), Advisor: Bruno Lindorfer

1. Conclusions and recommendations

1.1 The European Economic and Social Committee (EESC) asks the European Commission and Member States to urgently develop a plan to substantially increase the EU's single market autonomy regarding energy generation facilities, food and water production and the mining of the necessary raw materials, including sovereignty for the technologies needed. This EU sovereignty must consist of the respective R&D, material processing, design, manufacturing, installation, start-up and maintenance of the facilities within the EU single market so as to avoid energy poverty and unemployment among EU citizens and consumers. The most efficient preparedness for emergencies is based on resilience, be it technical or social. Continuous improvements in the resilience of energy systems towards natural, political or any other threats should be integrated into all energy policies.

1.2 The EESC recommends that the EU define short-term measures for building energy production facilities within the EU single market as a matter of urgency with a view to achieving the EU's goal of autonomy.

1.3 Widespread and long-lasting European energy shortages can be prevented by taking the following actions:
- strengthening and developing the European single market;
- enhancing cooperation and coordination with like-minded partners;
- pursuing an ambitious trade policy and the diversification of supply;
- tackling labour market mismatches;
- improving communication and raising awareness;
- accelerating innovation and digitalisation;
- facilitating access to finance;
- ensuring sufficient investments (to facilitate the green transition, etc.);
- ensuring that policies are realistic. For example, in the field of energy and climate we must reassess the Fit for 55 package in order to strike a balance between delivering on the goals for 2030 and 2050 and finding a pathway through this transition that is economically and socially bearable.

1.4 We therefore need to reconsider the timelines for the Green Deal and to implement realistic energy policies. The assessment procedures for the EU's Green Deal and energy policy should include not only the impact of the measures on the climate, but also the impact on the purchasing power of EU consumers and the impact on the competitiveness of the EU economy, thus safeguarding jobs in the EU.

1.5   No measures should be ruled out in the response to this crisis.

1.6   Implementing the EU SET plan (**S**trategic **E**nergy **T**echnology) and the REPowerEU plan:
- Improving energy efficiency and promoting circularity.
- Implementing the REPowerEU plan to end the EU's dependence on Russian fossil fuels.
- Increasing gas storage and coordinated refilling operations; monitoring and optimising electricity markets; channelling investments towards energy systems and enhancing connectivity in the immediate neighbourhood through Acer[1], Berec, ENTSO-G, ENTSO-E and the European Institute of Innovation and Technology's knowledge and innovation communities (KICs) on InnoEnergy, Raw materials and Manufacturing.

1.7   Consumers should invest in their own energy production and efficiency. This means that tax incentives are needed.

1.8   The EU should build new transport infrastructure for the transmission of energy and energy resources (pipeline from North Africa to Spain) and for renewable energy sources like hydrogen, biomethane and ammonia (Campfire).

1.9   Short-term measures:
- Safeguard other sources, especially oil, coal, gas, uranium, water, food and animal feed.
- Develop plans and concepts for saving and rationing energy in all 27 EU Member States:
  - Rationing should have clear priorities, e.g. negotiating plans for rationing and shutting off energy with energy-intensive industries, and negotiating new WTO trade agreements with new priorities for food, feed, water and sanitation;
  - Prioritising electricity and gas storage and supply for hospitals, medical care, emergency services and care for older and vulnerable people.
- Issue rules for safeguarding sufficient oil and gas reserve levels.
- Promote energy savings and new sources of energy.
- Step up EU R&D on energy research, especially alternative energies, fusion energy, energy storage, hydrogen and ammonia technologies, energy efficiency of energy-intensive industrial processes and consumer appliances.
- Accelerate public approval procedures for new projects that provide additional energy in the short and medium term, such as hydrogen unloading stations in EU harbours, pipelines and harbour facilities for re-gasification of liquified gas (LNG).

---

1   EU Agency for the Cooperation of Energy Regulators.

- Ask all firms in the EU that produce or provide products and services needed in emergency situations to secure their emergency electricity supply, update their emergency plans and organise periodic emergency training, etc. (for instance, companies involved in telecommunications and broadcasting, emergency services, public IT servers and electricity providers).

1.10 Medium- and long-term measures

1.10.1 The EESC asks the European Commission to develop plans and to undertake the following EU-wide coordinated measures and actions:
- Simplify and streamline EU regulations that slow down the procurement of critical energy infrastructure.
  - The new EU Water Framework Directive. Priority must be given to securing a quick energy supply, not to 10-year environmental impact assessments.
  - The EU's new supply chain regulation has to be simplified. The focus should be on securing a sustainable supply of critical raw materials and goods to the EU, not on overdesigned rules that dictate from which countries the EU is allowed to purchase materials (freezing 450 million Europeans in the coming winter).
- Reinforce production chains and transport systems to offset possible future disruption to the availability of critical raw materials for EU firms (industry and trade).
- Reduce dependence on imports of critical materials and prefabricated products.
- Focus on the EU's technological sovereignty/autonomy.
- Develop a cross-border power network infrastructure (380 kV or higher).
- Secure the production of transformers for electricity voltage change (high/low, AC/DC).
- Restart the thousands of energy production projects (hydropower, geothermal, hydro storage, etc.) that have been sidelined for years either because they had a bad pay-back ratio (due to cheap gas from Russia) or due to decades-long environmental impact assessments.
- Explore new exploitation technologies. There are several regions within the EU with substantial natural gas reservoirs which can be extracted using new technologies recently developed by European universities. In light of the EU's target for energy sovereignty/autonomy, the EU should seriously look into these new technologies and encourage the regions to try them.

1.10.2 Stepping up vocational training and skills for electricians and farmers and creating jobs in water stewardship are crucial in this transition.

1.10.3 Countries in Asia have substantially increased their numbers of physics (STEM graduates (STEM = **S**cience, **T**echnology, **E**ngineering, **M**athematics), ICT and engineering students, whereas the numbers of European STEMstudents remain stagnant.

1.10.4 In order for the EU to reach its technological sovereignty goals, hundreds of thousands of additional engineers are needed.

1.10.5 It is important to keep the purchasing power of EU citizens and consumers high by focusing on the EU's technology sovereignty and thus reducing its dependence on imports (technology and energy imports) and increasing the number of hightech jobs in Europe, rather than in Asia.

1.10.6 In an article published in May 2021[2], Dr Lukas Höber from the University of Leoben, Austria, calculated that to reach global decarbonisation goals (which most countries in the world pledged to achieve in the 1995 Paris Climate Agreement), around 7 million wind turbines in the 5 000 kW class would have to be built worldwide, along with large areas of photovoltaic systems.

1.10.7 The material requirements for the enormous number of wind turbines needed to reach the decarbonisation goals for electricity production exceed the annual global production of copper by a factor of 14 (25 million tons versus the 350 million tons needed), the annual global production of aluminium by a factor of 7.2, and the annual global production of the special steel needed for wind turbines by a factor of 3.9. Solar panels are mainly produced in China.

2. General comments

2.1 Definition of "emergency management": "emergency management" means the organisation and management of the resources and responsibilities for dealing with all humanitarian aspects of emergencies, i.e.:
- prevention
- preparedness
- response
- mitigation
- recovery.

2.2 As of March 2022, no one knows how long this brutal war will last, how much infrastructure will be destroyed, or how many millions of Ukrainian refugees will flee to the EU Member States – adding millions of new consumers to the single market.

2.3 The war in Ukraine will certainly have dramatic consequences for the EU, since the EU heavily relies on fossil fuels and raw materials imported from Russia and Ukraine.

---

2 https://www.profil.at/wissenschaft/erneuerbare-energien-warum-die-rechnung-nicht-aufgeht/401375021.

Investment into own mining and production facilities for power is urgently recommended to achieve autonomy – one of the EU's main goals.

2.4 In 2021, some European countries imported 100% of their natural gas imports from Russia, and some imported around 70% of their oil imports from Russia.

2.5 Consequently, the risk of massive job losses in the EU is increasing. According to EUROFER, the EU steel industry directly employs 330 000 highly-skilled people, and indirectly supports up to 2.2 million more. The aluminium, cement, paper and glass industries also directly and indirectly employ hundreds of thousands of people. Within the single market, the production facilities for energy production could provide hundreds of thousands of new wellpaid jobs, and therefore increase the purchasing power of EU consumers.

2.6 Food security: European countries will systematically seek to become less dependent on the supply of wheat from Ukraine and Russia. We need to look into fertiliser subsidies, set aside land for food and feed production and use agri-food waste to produce biogas.

3. **Disaster preparedness[3]**

3.1 Are our societies sufficiently prepared to manage and deal with situations that cause disruptions to the everyday functioning of society?

- Power outages (blackouts) caused by technical failures, cyberattacks, etc. that could affect:
  - communication systems;
  - sanitation systems, water supply and wastewater treatment;
  - industry business continuity.
- Electricity and gas rationing plans for EU consumers and EU industry. This risk has increased dramatically since the war in Ukraine.
- Disruption to the availability of raw materials due to production chain or transport system breakdowns (e.g. the traffic jam involving 400 large cargo ships in the Shanghai harbour in April 2022 due to Shanghai's COVID-19 lockdown).
- Cyber threats or incidents: how could the EU build business resilience and ensure business continuity to safeguard the supply needed for EU consumers?
- Other attacks: enterprises must be equipped to withstand and rapidly recover from attacks. Has the EU implemented solutions to ensure infrastructure availability and reliability?

---

3   https://ec.europa.eu/echo/what/humanitarian-aid/disaster-preparedness_de.

What are the challenges and costs for consumers and businesses in the event of such incidents, and how can they be mitigated to allow companies to continue their daily activities?

3.2 Emergencies and disasters emphasise the importance of the UN's 17 Sustainable Development Goals (SDGs)[4]. Disasters can be natural disasters[5], disasters caused by industrial or technological accidents (man-made machinery, ABC disasters), war and political and civil disasters[6], epidemics and famines, and the impact of food and feed production.

4.   Important organisations within the European Commission:
   – DG ECHO (European Civil Protection and Humanitarian Aid Operations)[7].
   – ERCC (Emergency Response Coordination Centre)[8].
   – UCP (Union Civil Protection) Knowledge Network[9].
   – European Union Civil Protection Mechanism (UCPM)[10].

5.   The five most serious emergencies and disasters for the EU's single market

5.1 Breakdown in the fossil energy production supply chain (coal, oil, natural gas, uranium). In 2021, fossil fuels made up approximately 80% of all primary energy used in the EU, the majority of which had been imported.

5.2 Power blackouts and subsequent communication breakdowns caused by technical failures, cyberwar or terror attacks. Renewable electric power production is erratic: the wind does not always blow and the sun does not always shine when the EU needs high amounts of energy, thus any increase in wind and PV-power generation capacities within the EU has to be accompanied by a buildup of huge energy storage facilities.

5.3 The ability to secure critical raw materials supplies (copper, lithium, cobalt, rare earth elements, etc.) through new EU single market strategies on mining, recycling, etc.

---

4   https://sdgs.un.org/goals.
5   https://www.conserve-energy-future.com/10-worst-natural-disasters.php.
6   https://www.samhsa.gov/find-help/disaster-distress-helpline/disaster-types/incidents-mass-violence.
7   https://ec.europa.eu/echo/index_de.
8   https://erccportal.jrc.ec.europa.eu/.
9   https://civil-protection-knowledge-network.europa.eu/.
10 https://ec.europa.eu/echo/what/civil-protection/eu-civil-protection-mechanism_de.

5.4 The ability to secure a competitive single market for half-finished product supplies (e.g. the EU auto industry has seen a severe shortage of Ukrainian-produced cable looms since the war in Ukraine started).

5.5 Massive fossil fuel supplies are urgently needed until a sufficient amount of production facilities for renewable energy installations has been built in the EU.

5.6 The Russian invasion of Ukraine has shone an unforgiving light on the extreme vulnerability of the EU's energy system, and its lack of own production facilities within the single market.

6. Response

6.1 Given the magnitude of the EU's energy consumption, the EU's green transition will take roughly two decades. The Council meeting in Versailles recommended that the transition be accelerated, which would prove a very challenging task.

6.2 The major bottleneck preventing a faster transfer is not about money, but rather the materials needed for the approximately 700 000 large 5 MW wind turbines needed across the EU, and the millions of photovoltaic installations, fusion energy, waterpower and energy storage facilities. In addition, geothermal facilities and hydrogen and CO_2 storage facilities will have to be built. In order to distribute the massively increased amount of decentralised electric power generated, highvoltage and medium-voltage power transmission lines will have to be expanded on a colossal scale.

6.3 Each of these 700 000 large 5 MW wind turbines (which typically produce 12.5 GWh of electric energy p.a.) has a height of around 200 metres, a foundation of around 2000 tons of reinforced concrete, requires approximately 600 tons of special steel, 20 tons of copper and a supply of very scarce rare earth materials which have to be imported mainly from China or Russia. If these tons of materials required are multiplied by the approximately 700 000 wind turbines needed within the EU, it becomes clear that we will need huge amounts of concrete, steel, copper and other materials – the production of which would emit huge additional amounts of CO_2. For rare earth elements (for the electric generators and batteries), neodymium, dysprosium, etc., the shortage problem is even more dire, and would be very difficult to solve by 2050.

7. Mitigation

7.1 To achieve the Green Deal targets, Germany alone has to build approximately 70 000 new large 5 MW wind turbines by 2050 (or even faster). This means commissioning 2 500 new wind turbines per year, or seven every day until 2050 in Germany alone. In 2021, Germany built approximately 450 new wind turbines. Therefore, if Germany continues to build wind turbines at 2021 rates, building the 70 000 wind turbines needed for the Green Deal would take 160 years.

7.2 In addition to the material shortages for building the 700 000 wind turbines, in the EU there is also a massive shortage of electricians and engineers to implement the Green Deal by 2050. Austria, for example, has ambitious expansion targets for photovoltaic systems by 2040; however, according to Austrian experts, there is a shortage of thousands of qualified electricians to install the PV systems needed to reach this target.

7.3 To summarise, many engineers claim that achieving the Green Deal goals by 2050 is very challenging and perhaps not even feasible, and not for lack of money but due to materials shortages (rare earth elements, copper, steel, etc.), and a massive shortage of electricians and engineers in the EU.

8. Prevention

8.1 Many energy-intensive industries are to be converted to renewable green hydrogen or ammonia produced by renewable electric power by 2050, including the steel industry, the chemical industry and the cement industry. Many people are unaware that transitioning all these energy-intensive industries requires approximately 10 times more renewable electric power than the transition to e-mobility and decarbonising the steel industry.

8.2 Iron and steel production accounts for a quarter of all global industrial CO_2 emissions. Around 1 870 million tons of steel were produced worldwide in 2020; approximately 57% of that was produced in China, and 7% in the EU. Of the 1 870 million tons of steel produced globally, around 1 300 million tons (65%) are made via the integrated blast furnace route, where iron ore is reduced with coke, generating very high CO2 emissions (approximately 1.4 tons of CO2 per ton of steel).

8.3 Within the EU 27 Member States, approximately 150 million tons of steel are produced p.a., approximately 90 million tons thereof via the blast furnace route. To switch the production of these 90 million tons of pig iron (reduced in the blast furnace with coke) to renewable hydrogen green iron, around 360 TWh p.a. of renewable electricity would be needed (by 2050). 360 TWh p.a. is a huge amount of renewable energy! It is more renewable electricity than that needed for the electrification of all passenger cars in the whole EU. No less than 30 000 large wind turbines will be needed to produce this renewable electricity for the EU's steel industry.

8.4 Looking at the European Union, electricity production in 2019 was approx. 2 904 TWh, only around 35% of which was from renewable sources. However, about 38% (1 112 TWh) was produced from fossil fuels and around 26% from nuclear power (765 TWh). Only 13% was produced from wind power, 12% from hydropower plants, 4% from solar power plants, 4% from bioenergy and 2% from geothermal supplies. The bulk of renewable electricity generation in the European Union in 2019 (1 005 TWh) was from wind power (367 TWh, 42% of all renewables). A further 39% was generated by hydropower plants (345 TWh), 12% from solar power plants (125 TWh) and the remaining 6% from bioenergy (55 TWh).

8.5 The expansion of pumped storage hydropower plants has to be supported immediately.

8.6 Hydropower must be moved up the energy and climate policy agenda. Sustainably developed hydropower plants need to be recognised as renewable energy sources. Governments should include large and small hydropower in their long-term deployment targets, energy plans and renewable energy incentive schemes, on a par with variable renewables.

8.7 Priorities have switched from the environment, price and security of supply to security of supply, price and the environment.

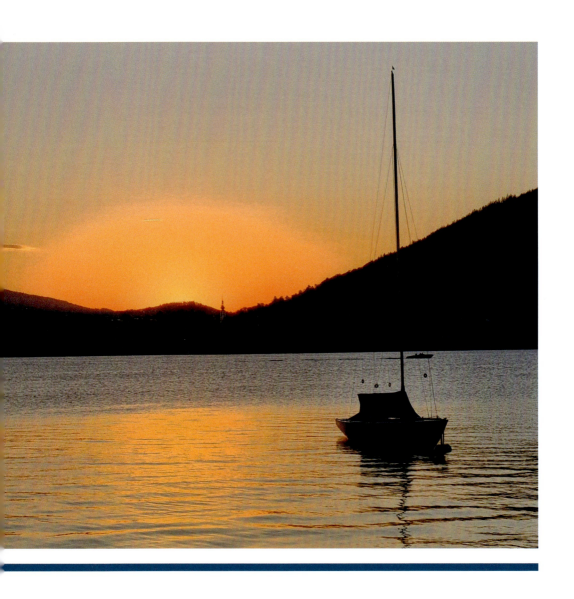

INT/924

OPINION EUROPEAN ECONOMIC AND SOCIAL COMMITTEE
A NEW EUROPEAN RESEARCH AREA FOR RESEARCH AND
INNOVATION

Paul Rübig

1.   Conclusions and recommendations

1.1   The European Economic and Social Committee (EESC) welcomes the new vision for, and the renewal of, the ERA agenda. The new ERA is not just "more of the same", but is a real "New Deal" for the EU's Research, Technology and Innovation (RTI).

1.2   The EESC strongly welcomes the focus on rapidly translating R&I results into sustainable business, as outlined in the document. Safeguarding a just transition process is one of the most important elements to ensure that R&I supports the economy and employment in the EU.

1.3   The EESC strongly advocates the need for new governance in the research area in order to remove administrative and regulatory barriers to innovation.

1.4   The EESC welcomes the fact that the new ERA document is overall in line with and supports the UN Sustainable Development Goals (SDG). While fostering the transition towards a more resilient European economy, an inclusive recovery leaving no European behind is essential in the process of moving towards a sustainable European economy[1].

1.5   The EESC would like to point out that an intelligent blending of R&D instruments at all levels (regional, national, global level, EU level) is important. R&D and innovation should be promoted by making use of the large EU structural funds, too, as well as through direct and indirect measures (e.g. tax incentives) for R&D.

1.6   The EESC suggests that the following key sectors and technologies are vital for the prosperity of the EU:
  – Digital business models;
  – Technologies for manufacturing goods and food;
  – Clinical research, pharmaceutical and biotechnological sector;
  – Space technologies;
  – Clean water and sanitation.

1.7   The EESC notes that research in the social sciences and humanities is very important for the complex renewal of the ERA agenda.

---

1   EESC proposals for post-COVID-19 crisis reconstruction and recovery: "The EU must be guided by the principle of being considered a community of common destiny", OJ C 311, 18.9.2020, p. 1, pt. 5.3.1.

1.8   The EESC would like to emphasise the fact that EU research lags behind in patent performance. Asia has increased its share of global patent applications. In 2019, Asia submitted 65% of global patent applications. Europe's share of patents has decreased and is now only 11.3% of global patent applications.

1.9   Numerous studies have shown that the EU is lagging behind the US and Asia in entrepreneurial culture. Entrepreneurial culture needs to be addressed in education, including higher education. Entrepreneurial culture shall therefore be relevant throughout the whole process, from innovation in basic research and applied research to marketing of a new technology.

1.10   The EIC and the EIT, with its KICs, are considered valuable partners and tools in this "acceleration of R&I translation" and in redirecting the focus of the EU's R&I towards the generation of breakthrough innovations that address concrete needs of citizens and business, particularly in relation to major societal challenges. The EIC accelerator offers substantial EU funds for innovative European startups with high growth potential, whereas the EIT by definition pursues research excellence for technologypush innovations in its KICs; thus both the EIC and the EIT are important partners regarding the acceleration of R&I translation.

1.11   The EESC underlines the need to incorporate the principle of scientific and ethical integrity, so as to prevent losses in terms of human health, money, and scientific failure.

1.12   Europe is especially lagging behind the US and Asia regarding the speed of transferring R&D results into innovative products and services. Thus, the EESC encourages the Commission to aim in its RTI policy on "excellence" as well as "speed" at the same time.

1.13   The EESC suggests that the European Commission should aim, in its new R&I strategy, for well-balanced portfolios:
- of high-tech industrial production as well as service industry R&D/R&I;
- market-pull innovations (demand-driven innovation) as well as technology-push innovations.

2.   General comments

2.1   The EESC welcomes the fact that a new vision for and the renewal of the ERA agenda are key elements in the document. The document thus proves that the new ERA is not just "more of the same", but is a real "New Deal" for the EU's RTI. A key aspect of the "New Deal" is the objective of massively increasing the impact of innovation on the economy and society. With this "New Deal", the EU-27 is definitively committed to stopping the ongoing process of losing ground to China and South Korea in basic research as well as in applied research, patent applications, hightech products and services. The "New Deal" aims to even better educate and train European citizens in all kinds of R&D, innovation and entrepreneurship, and thus to fully unleash the innovation power of European society.

2.2 The EESC welcomes the approach of the European Commission to increase the impact of innovation on the economy and society. The EESC emphasises that organised civil society is a catalyst for social innovation. The participation of civil society is needed now more than ever – and true social innovation only happens with when organised civil society is involved[2].

2.3 Asia, especially China and Korea, has massively improved its performance in RTI within the last 20 years. China has not only increased its share of spending on R&D from 0.55% (1995) to 2.2% (2018), but has also outperformed the EU in the total budget spent on R&D, spending USD 496 billion in 2017, while the EU spent USD 430 billion. According to the 2020 EU Industrial R&D Investment Scoreboard, from 2018 to 2019, EU companies increased R&D by 5.6%, US companies by 10.8% and Chinese companies by 21.0%.

2.4 The OECD's Science, Technology and Industry Scoreboard reports show, among other things, that the EU is especially lagging behind in digital service businesses and what are known as breakthrough technology-push innovations. The EESC advocates a European path of digitalisation by seizing the opportunities for the economy while safeguarding societal values and fundamental rights. A human-centred focus in all Commission initiatives is very much welcome with a view to developing a European approach to progress[3].

2.5 Promoting the development of breakthrough innovations[4] while safeguarding a just transition process is one of the key challenges in the near future.

2.6 The EESC fully supports putting one clear focus on the Twin Transition, i.e. the Digital Transition and the Green Deal.

---

2   EESC proposals for post-COVID-19 crisis reconstruction and recovery: "The EU must be guided by the principle of being considered a community of common destiny",OJ C 311, 18.9.2020, p. 1, pt. 6.8.

3   OJ C 364, 28.10.2020, p. 101.

4   Clayton M. Christensen, The Innovator's Dilemma – When New Technologies Cause Great Firms to Fail, 2016.

2.7 The EESC welcomes efforts to ensure that R&I results are rapidly translated into sustainable business. Safeguarding a just transition process, i.e. towards a greener/climate-friendly Europe, a fair digital future, with respect for workers' rights and positions, as outlined in the document, is one of the most important elements to ensure that R&I supports the economy and employment in the EU.

2.8 The EESC welcomes the fact that the new ERA document is overall in line with and supports the SDGs. While fostering the transition towards a more resilient European economy, an inclusive recovery leaving no European behind is essential in the process of moving towards a sustainable European economy[5].

2.9 The EESC would like to point out that an intelligent blending of R&D instruments at all levels (regional, national level, EU level) is important. R&D and innovation should be promoted by making use of the large EU structural funds, too, as well as through direct and indirect measures (e.g. tax incentives) for R&D.

3. **The European Research Area in a new context**

3.1 As pointed out in our general comments, the EESC clearly thinks that, if the EU's RTI strategy remains "more of the same", it will continue to lose ground in the global RTI competition, especially against China, Korea and the USA.

3.2 The EESC underlines the need to incorporate the principle of scientific and ethical integrity, so as to prevent losses in terms of human health, money, and scientific failure.

3.3 The EESC encourages the European Commission to design a "New Deal" RTI agenda for the EU.

3.4 State-of-the-art, efficiently managed R&I infrastructures are one important key issue for this acceleration of R&I translation.

3.5 The day-to-day management of these R&I infrastructures could be professionalised in the EESC's view. Utilisation of some of these expensive R&I infrastructures is relatively low: some have a utilisation of less than 25% of annual working hours.

3.6 The EESC welcomes the EC's Open Science Initiatives (EOSC).

---

5 EESC proposals for post-COVID-19 crisis reconstruction and recovery: "The EU must be guided by the principle of being considered a community of common destiny",OJ C 311, 18.9.2020, p. 1, pt. 5.3.1.

3.7 The EESC agrees that the technologies mentioned in the document are very important, strategic key technologies for the EU, and proposes that the following key technologies and sectors be added:

- Digital business models;
- Technologies for manufacturing goods and food;
- Clinical research, pharmaceutical and biotechnological sector;
- Space technologies;
- Clean water and sanitation.

3.8 Digital business models are currently the fastest growing businesses in the globe and will continue to be in the years to come. One just has to look at e-commerce (e.g. Amazon), Industry 4.0, e-banking, e-gaming, digital social networks (e.g. Facebook), e-security, etc.

3.9 The EESC notes that research in the social sciences and humanities is very important for the complex renewal of the ERA agenda.

3.10 The EESC notes that EU research lags behind in patent performance. Asia has increased its share of global patent applications. In 2019, Asia submitted 65% of global patent applications. Europe's share of patents has decreased and is now 11.3% of global patent applications.

3.11 Other important R&I topics include (but are not limited to) manufacturing of goods (which has always been and still is a stronghold of the EU), IT, software and AI, and medium tech.

3.12 Most of the jobs within the EU still are in medium tech (which, similarly, has always been a stronghold of the EU). High tech is of course important, but there is a lot of growth potential and job potential in medium tech too.

3.13 The coronavirus crisis is a severe challenge for mankind and all possible measures should be taken to develop vaccines and treatments for COVID-19. This crisis has exposed several issues that need to be addressed to prevent similar pandemics in the future, not least as regards our relationship with the natural world and animals. European R&I must play an important role in identifying, researching and solving those issues. On the other hand, the crisis should not be the only guideline for the EU's long-term R&I strategy.

3.14 Numerous studies have shown that the EU is lagging behind the US and Asia in entrepreneurial culture. Entrepreneurial culture needs to be addressed in education, including higher education. Entrepreneurial culture shall therefore be relevant throughout the whole process, from innovation in basic research and applied research to marketing of a new technology. Entrepreneurial culture must be a key competence in all of the EU's RTI and thus, of course, in the new ERA too.

4. The vision: a stronger European Research Area for the future

4.1 The communication devotes a number of paragraphs to new common technology roadmaps, a New Industrial Strategy and key future technologies for the Commission. The EESC, again, would like to point out that all these topics need to be seen in close connection with the SDGs. In other words, R&D needs to be pushed in particular within the new ERA and common technology roadmaps, where any of the 17 areas of the SDGs can be supported. The EESC is convinced that a constructive social and civic dialogue at all levels will contribute to a successful implementation of the strategy.

4.2 The EESC appreciates the strengthening of RTI cooperation within the EU. Any EU Member State alone is simply too small to compete with the large research nations such as the USA or China. The individual Member States lack "economies of scale", which are very important especially for large breakthrough innovations. Europe's achievements in science and technology have been significant and research and development efforts form an integral part of the European economy. Europe has been the home of some of the most prominent researchers in various scientific disciplines, notably physics, mathematics, chemistry and engineering. Scientific research in Europe is supported by industry, by the European universities and by several scientific institutions. The output from European scientific research consistently ranks among the world's best. While cooperation is one key element in efficient innovation to generate new products and services, competition is the major driving force for innovation in the global economy. Thus the EESC recommends a well-balanced portfolio of cooperation as well as competition between the Member States in the EU's "New Deal" for RTI.

4.3 The EIC and the EIT with its KICs, are considered valuable partners and tools in this "acceleration of R&I translation" and in redirecting the focus of the EU's R&I towards the generation of breakthrough innovations that address concrete needs of citizens and business, particularly in relation to major societal challenges.

5. Translating R&I results into the economy

5.1 The communication states that "The EU is lagging behind its main global competitors in business R&D intensity, in particular in high-tech sectors, and in scaling-up innovative SMEs with negative effects on productivity and competitiveness. (...) Unlocking investment in innovation in business, services as well as in the public sector is critical to reversing this trend, as well as to reinforce Europe's industrial and technological sovereignty. The EU needs to make full use of its excellent research and innovation results to support the green and digital transition of the EU economy". The EESC shares this position, but wants to stress that the digital transition in particular needs a responsible RTI approach. The EESC reiterates its full support for the EU's strategy of seeking trustworthy and human-centric artificial intelligence (AI), and reiterates its call for a "human-in-command" approach to AI, as called for since its first opinion on AI in 2017[6].

5.2 Europe is especially lagging behind the US and Asia regarding the speed of transferring R&D results into innovative products and services. Thus, the EESC encourages the Commission to aim in its RTI policy on "excellence" as well as "speed" at the same time.

5.3 The EESC certainly recognises that the communication acknowledges that R&I translation into viable products and the chain of innovation need attention. However, most actions and measures proposed in the document still focus on the input side of the chain of innovation (higher education, research careers for talented people, more money for public and basic research, etc.).

5.4 The EESC encourages the Commission to aim for a well-balanced equilibrium between focusing on the input side of the chain of innovation and the output side.

5.5 The EESC encourages the Commission to further stimulate market-pull innovations by, for example:
- promoting lead user concepts;
- investing in systematic social innovation studies to anticipate early appreciation and acceptance of new products and services by society.

6.   Service industries

6.1 Industrial production processes can be highly automated, such that they can produce very high batch sizes with a small share of labour costs and globally competitive production costs, even with Europe's high hourly wages. Regarding service industries, this situation is more complicated. Digital service business models, too, can be highly automated. Services to individuals, like hair-cutting, massages, etc., however, cannot be automated. For all these reasons, the EU would be well advised to aim, in its new R&I strategy, for a well balanced portfolio of high-tech industrial production and service industries.

---

6   OJ C 288, 31.8.2017, p. 1.

7. Deepening the Framework for Research Careers

7.1 The EESC welcomes the measures proposed in the communication to enhance the technological and scientific excellence and the mobility of young researchers, but encourages the Commission to step up measures regarding enhancing the entrepreneurship of young researchers and innovators as well. This would include better career prospects for researchers as well as higher salaries, especially for researchers at the beginning of their careers. Furthermore, connecting universities with economic entities to ensure the transformation of innovation into marketable products seems to be fruitful. The EESC proposes establishing a single register of EU researchers and innovators with basic professional research data to connect EU researchers and innovators more closely.

7.2 Key competences and key innovative cultures, new learning and teaching technologies, personalised training.

7.2.1 The EESC would once again like to point out that it is not only key strategic technologies that are very important, but that key competences of employees and innovative cultures within all EU enterprises are also very important if the EU is to prosper.

7.2.2 The following element is especially important for the new ERA agenda, the new R&I agenda and the new "Pact for Research and Innovation in Europe": fostering an innovative culture and a culture of entrepreneurship within EU enterprises, for the management as well as for all employees, for example by offering appropriate training courses, etc. to employees.

8. Citizens' engagement

8.1 The EESC agrees with the statement in the communication that "The engagement of citizens, local communities and civil society will be at the core of the new ERA to achieve greater societal impact and increased trust in science". The EESC explains its support for the European Commission's approach which is based on the idea that "research organisations and industry should involve citizens in technology choices".

8.2 The social partners and civil society organisations such as consumer organisations, NGOs, etc. should be involved as active partners in European R&I processes and projects, in particular when the research affects or impacts the people or cause they represent. Involving these partners at an early stage will promote engagement, understanding, ownership and acceptance of the innovation, and support the just transition processes that are necessary, especially for breakthrough innovations. It will also help researchers understand the impact of their innovations on society at large and help them address potential negative impacts at an early stage in the process. For this reason, the EESC has also been calling for a multidisciplinary approach in certain research areas, where there is an impact on multiple research areas. One of these areas is again AI, where the EESC has been calling for the involvement of the humanities, law, economics, ethics, psychology, etc. in the R&I of AI, beyond the mere technical element[7].

8.3   The EU's economy relies heavily on exports of its goods and services.

8.4   Technology choices should thus be based on EU citizens' preferences for goods and services, but also on those of the rest of the 7.8 billion people in the world. The EESC calls on the Commission to particularly promote R&I in reaching the UN SDGs.

8.5   As pointed out in our general comments, the importance of RTI needs to be better communicated to politicians, the media and society.

8.6   It is therefore also important to develop smart means and strategies for communicating the importance of RTI, but also its results, in the context of the communication and the new EU RTI strategy.

9.   Governance of the new ERA

9.1   The EESC agrees that a transparent monitoring system (ERA Scoreboard) will be essential in order to monitor the EU's performance in the global RTI competition. The EESC advocates the need for new governance in the research area in order to remove administrative and regulatory barriers to innovation.

---

7   OJ C 288, 31.8.2017, p. 1.

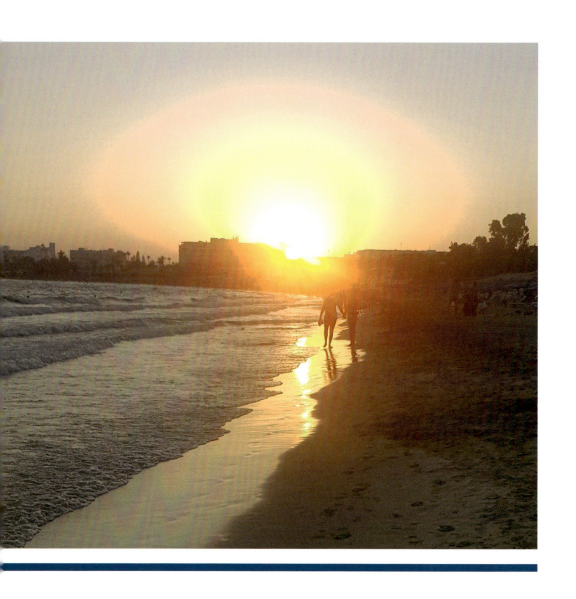

INT/967

OPINION EUROPEAN ECONOMIC AND SOCIAL COMMITTEE
EUROPEAN MISSIONS

Paul Rübig, Małgorzata Anna Bogusz (Co-Author)

1.   Conclusions and recommendations

1.1   While the EESC feels that the five missions presented in the communication are high priorities for the EU, the EESC also considers the five challenges and objectives listed below to be very important for Europe.

Develop and pursue missions and measures to:
1. keep up with the USA and Asia in global competition in the areas of research, technology and innovation (RTI);
2. cope with the challenges linked to the EU's ageing society;
3. define strategies for the successful integration of the high number of migrants coming into the EU;
4. improve emergency preparedness;
5. cope with the needs of patients with non-communicable diseases (NCD) impacted by the COVID-19 pandemic, especially those who suffer from cardio-vascular disease.

1.2   The communication lists and addresses five priority EU Missions:
1. Adaptation to climate change;
2. Cancer;
3. Restore our ocean and waters by 2030, including sanitation;
4. 100 climate-neutral and smart cities by 2030, including smart villages;
5. A soil deal for Europe.

1.3   The EESC strongly supports the idea of empowering 150 climate benchmark regions throughout Europe. However, this will require a huge R&D budget. The EESC therefore strongly recommends increasing the portion of the EU regional budgets earmarked for R&D from the current figure of 5% to a minimum of 10%.

1.4   The EESC welcomes the fact that the EU is focusing on fighting cancer as one of the most important health issues, and wishes to encourage the EU institutions to undertake similar steps with respect to cardio-vascular diseases – the number one killer of European citizens and around the world.

2.   General comments

2.1   EU Missions will deliver results through a new role for research and innovation under the Horizon Europe programme, combined with a coordinated, all-in approach, and a new relationship with citizens. They will fully mobilise and engage with public and private actors, such as EU Member States, regional and local authorities, research institutes, entrepreneurs, and public and private investors, all to create real and lasting impact.

2.2   The EESC would like to highlight that the competitiveness of Europe's industry is very important in order to achieve the EU's Missions. The EESC therefore welcomes the reference to the new industrial competitiveness agenda. At the same time, the EESC underlines the importance of considering the impact on EU citizens and encourages the Commission to strongly link activities to social policies and the European Pillar of Social Rights, taking in particular into account the special needs of elderly and vulnerable EU citizens.

2.3   The EESC wishes to highlight that, while the major focus of the European Missions is delivering impact for the EU through a new and greater role for research and innovation, the economic dimension (global competition, high quality jobs etc.) as well as the social dimension also have to play a major role within these European Missions. As far as the social dimension is concerned, the EESC would like to emphasise that besides the importance of social rights and the safeguarding of the social security and fair working conditions for all employees, special attention has to be paid to the special needs of vulnerable groups in the EU (elderly people, sick people etc.)

2.4   The EESC very much welcomes the fact that R&I is clearly seen as the core issue of the EU Missions document. The EESC is convinced that complex challenges lying ahead of the EU can be addressed primarily through R&I.

2.5   The EESC adopted its opinion on *A new ERA for Research and Innovation* in March 2021[1], an opinion on the *Pact for Research and Innovation in Europe*, in February 2022[2], and an opinion on *An intellectual property action plan to support the EU´s recovery and resilience*[3]. The present opinion should be seen in close conjunction with these three recent EESC opinions.

2.6   The EESC fully agrees that, due to the current challenges, "continuing with the status quo is not an option". Europe needs "a new kind of research and innovation policy": if the EU continues with more of the same of its "old" R&I policy, it will not be able to tackle the huge challenges facing it, namely fierce competition from Asia. The EESC pointed this out very clearly in its opinion on *A new ERA for Research and Innovation*.

2.7   Regarding enterprises, the communication states that the European Missions will fully mobilise and engage with public and private stakeholders, such as the EU Member

---

1   OJ C 220, 9.6.2021, p. 79
2   EESC opinion (adopted on 23.02.2022)
3   OJ C 286, 16.7.2021, p. 59

States, regional and local authorities, research institutes, entrepreneurs and public and private investors, EU citizens and civil society, all to create real and lasting impact, taking into account industry and businesses, particularly MSMEs.

2.8 The competitiveness of the EU's industry regarding technologies for the decarbonisation of electricity generation as well as of other CO_2 intensive industries is a decisive factor in achieving the EU's Mission 1 – "Adaptation to climate change". If the EU does not succeed, it will lose millions of job in these industries.

2.9 The EESC also fully agrees that the EU Missions must be fully consistent with the United Nations sustainable development goals (SDGs).

2.10 While the EESC feels that the five missions are high priorities for the EU, it considers the additional five challenges and missions listed in chapter 4 to also be very important for Europe.

2.11 The EESC recommends that the European Commission also prioritise missions and measures that generate new, highquality jobs, business, income, wealth and a high quality of living for EU citizens, such as maintaining the competitiveness of Europe's technological products against increasingly fierce global competition (especially with China, South Korea, etc.).

2.12 A substantial amount of Europe's jobs and wealth stems from exports of Europe's technological products (cars, machinery, materials, etc.). Another important source of new jobs in Europe are MSMEs, innovative startups, scaleups and higher education.

3. Specific comments

3.1 Mission 1 – **Adaptation to Climate Change**

3.1.1 Climate change is one of the biggest challenges for humanity in the 21st century. Policy makers will need to anticipate the changes ahead in order to protect the sectors and groups most at risk, also considering employment.

3.1.2 With almost all Green Deal measures, prices for electricity, fuel, domestic heating etc. increase for EU citizens. These price increases have a particularly high impact on the hundreds of millions of people within the EU Member States with low and medium incomes and vulnerable people in general, which often are low-income EU citizens.

This means that all Green Deal measures have a significant social impact and must be handled carefully. They must increase prosperity instead of sidelining those who need support to tackle the change.

3.1.3   Examples of new technologies that will certainly play a very important role in reducing CO_2 emissions include:
- decarbonisation of electricity generation;
- decarbonisation of CO_2-emitting industries, e.g. the steel industry, the cement industry, etc.;
- carbon capture and storage (CCS) and, for example, sewage treatment plants;
- storage of electric power on a very large scale for low specific costs;
- e-mobility;
- smart grids and high-voltage power grids;
- smart cities, etc.

3.1.4   These technologies are easy to list on paper, but implementing them is undoubtedly a huge challenge, given the scale needed for all 27 EU Member States as well as globally.

3.1.5   One key issue in this global competition regarding new technologies will be the availability of a high number of researchers and engineers. This is definitely a huge challenge for Europe. Countries in Asia, have increased the number of students in physics, ICT and engineering massively over the last 20 years, whereas numbers have been more or less stagnant in Europe. The European Missions should not only promote an increase in the number of these students, but the EU should promote a change in the current "brain drain" of highly qualified people into a "brain gain" for the EU.

3.1.6   The EESC strongly recommends that the Commission define measures to substantially improve basic skills as well as increase the number of students in physics, ICT and engineering, and also in medicine and pharmacology in Europe in the next 20 years. Without this engineering brain trust, Europe will continue to fall behind in all technologies needed to fight climate change.

3.2   Mission 2 – **Cancer**

3.2.1   The EU 27 is witnessing steadily increasing numbers of cancer cases. The EU 27 must work together on improving diagnosis, therapy, access to personalised medicines, treatment and prevention – as was already emphasised in the EESC's opinion on *Europe's Beating Cancer Plan* in June 2021[4]. Therefore, the EESC welcomes the fact

---

4   OJ C 341, 24.8.2021, p.76.

that research for cancer prevention and cure has been indicated as one of the five EU Missions.

3.2.2 The EESC wants to clearly emphasise that one of the toughest challenges will be to level out the disparities in access to cancer treatment between individual countries. The EESC advises that a special focus has to be put on vulnerable groups within the EU.

3.2.3 As was already described in the EESC opinion on *Europe's Beating Cancer Plan*, access to the most innovative therapies and the introduction of vaccination campaigns that will enable us to reduce the number of cancers caused by viral infections play a unique role here.

3.2.4 The EESC wants to emphasise the need of a more active approach towards prevention of occupational cancer. As it was stressed in the opinion *Europe's Beating Cancer Plan*, the EESC calls for more research into occupational exposure to carcinogens, mutagens and endocrine disruptors and the causes of occupational cancers.

3.2.5 The EESC wants to stress that social partners, patient advocacy groups and civil society organisations have an indispensable role to play by disseminating best practices and providing relevant information – about the causes of cancer and about special issues relating to, for example, gender or vulnerable groups,

3.3 Mission 3 – **Restore our Ocean and Waters by 2030**

3.3.1 Clean water is of major importance for EU citizens, agriculture and for its fishing industry. Again, research and clean water technologies, including waste water mining, sanitation and sewage treatment are key for this mission.

3.3.2 Furthermore, access to clean water still is an issue for many citizens. The EESC encourages the Commission to legally implement the human rights to water and sanitation.

3.4 Mission 4 – **100 Climate-Neutral and Smart Cities by 2030**

3.4.1 More than 65% of the global population lives in large cities, and this percentage is growing. These large cities impose growing challenges in terms of infrastructure (water supply and sewage, transport, energy supply, etc.) and quality of life. Many of the challenges can only be solved by research and hightech solutions. Much more highly-skilled engineers will be needed in the future to plan these hightech smart cities and villages.

3.4.2 The proportion of older people in cities is growing fast ("ageing society"). Older people and vulnerable people have needs differing from young people: they need more medical care, social care, etc. Due to the demographic shift in society, there will not be enough young people to provide all these services in the near future, which mean that some of these services for older people will have to be taken over by smart solutions (e.g. robots).

3.4.3 Many emergencies within recent years have shown that modern societies are relatively vulnerable, thus increasing "emergency preparedness" through R&D is very important:
- disasters in the nuclear power plants in Fukushima, Chernobyl, Three Mile Island etc.;
- electricity blackouts and communication blackouts;
- shortages of and steep price increases in all energy sources, including natural gas;
- thunderstorms and massive floods, with many hundreds of people killed;
- pandemics, such as the COVID-19 pandemic, Zika and future pandemics;
- cyberattacks (with the massively growing digitalisation of everything in public life, private life and business, the threat of cyberattacks is growing rapidly).

3.4.4 Eastern and southern Europe barely escaped a huge power blackout on 8 January 2021. The root cause for the increasing vulnerability of Europe's power supply is the increasing share of unpredictable and unplannable renewable electric power, such as wind turbines and solar power. Europe is not very well prepared for blackouts: in the event of a blackout, the energy supply to private households and industry breaks down immediately, communication breaks down within minutes or hours, the supply of drinking water breaks down within a short time etc. Recovering from a major electricity blackout is not an easy task.

3.5 Mission 5 – **A Soil Deal for Europe**

3.5.1 Along with clean water, as mentioned above, healthy soil to grow the basic ingredients for food is one of the most important resources for all living creatures, including humans and animals. The global population is growing: by the end of the century we will need to feed approximately 10 billion people on a sustainable basis. Conventional food and farming are one of the major sources of the greenhouse gases CO_2 and methane. This means that a large amount of R&D is needed to research and develop climate neutral agriculture for the sustainable production of food for the 10 billion people living on the globe. Currently, approximately 10% of the EU's budget for agriculture and farming is spent on R&D; the EESC recommends increasing this figure to a minimum of 20% to increase R&D for new, sustainable farming technologies, including in particular robotics in farming technologies and food.

4. Five additional missions

4.1 While the EESC considers the five missions listed in the communication to be high priorities for the EU, it feels that the 5 challenges and missions described below are also of high importance.

4.2 Additional EU Mission 1 – **Keeping up with the USA and Asia in the global competition in RTI**

4.2.1 It is important to define and pursue missions and measures to prevent the EU falling behind Asia in research, technology, innovation (RTI) and patents, especially in comparison with China and South Korea. It is a fact that the EU has been falling behind China and South Korea regarding RTI at an increasing pace since approximately 2000[5].

4.2.2 If the EU continues to fall behind the USA and Asia in RTI, Europe will lose millions of jobs and considerable wealth in the long run (20 to 50 years). The shortfall of the EU27 really is critical, especially in key enabling technologies (KETs) and future emerging technologies (FETs), such as artificial intelligence, machine learning, deep learning, robotics, genetic engineering, communication technologies (e.g. 5G), computer chip manufacturing, manufacturing of key components for e-mobility (e.g. batteries, fuel cells and hydrogen), etc. New materials have always been and will always be a driver for innovation: for example, graphene innovation and its industrial upscaling has substantial potential for research and innovation for Europe.

4.3. Additional EU Mission 2 – **Coping with the challenges of the EU's ageing society**

4.3.1 EU society is ageing fast, and this will create several new challenges for all EU Member States.

4.3.2 Older people and vulnerable people have different needs from young people: they need more and new medicine (for dementia, Alzheimer's disease, etc.), more medical care, more social care, and special training and education, especially designed for older and vulnerable people, etc.

4.3.3 Research and innovation (in medicine, pharmaceuticals, social sciences, engineering sciences, special training courses etc.) will undoubtedly play a major role in helping cope with the EU's ageing society.

---

5   Details can be read e.g. in the OECD STI-Reports 2015 and 2017.

4.3.4   Society as a whole needs an ambitious European care strategy.

4.4   Additional EU Mission 3 – **Strategies for the successful integration of the high number of migrants coming into the EU**

4.4.1   The EU needs to develop missions and measures for the integration of this high number of migrants into the EU Member States. Since the EU is a rapidly ageing society, it needs more young, well-educated people. Thus, innovative concepts for educating and training migrants are needed. Socioeconomic research can help develop a better understanding of what is needed for the successful integration of these millions of people.

4.5   Additional EU Mission 4 – **Emergency Preparedness**

4.5.1   Emergency preparedness involves developing and pursuing missions and measures to safeguard a stable energy supply and to avoid electricity blackouts, while decarbonising the EU's energy system. In this regard, see point 3.4.4, which addresses the issue of emergency preparedness, especially the challenge of electricity blackouts and communication blackouts. Again, research and innovation, primarily in the engineering sciences, is the key to addressing these challenges.

4.5.2   Other emergency challenges include floods, droughts, pandemics, but also economic emergency situations, e. g. the blocking of global supply chains (e.g. the blocking of the Suez Canal in 2021, etc.)

4.6   Additional EU Mission 5 – **Coping with the needs of patients with non-communicable diseases (NCD) impacted by the COVID-19 pandemic, especially those suffering from cardiovascular disease – the number one cause of death of European citizens and globally.**

4.6.1   After the pandemic, more focus is needed on non-communicable diseases (NCD). In the EU there are 60 million people living with cardio-vascular diseases (CVD) – it is the number one killer of European citizens. In non-COVID-19 years, CVD is the most common cause of preventable deaths in the EU. During the pandemic, many of these patients have been diagnosed too late or did not have a chance to be diagnosed at all.

4.6.2   We should look into the health equity dimension in the EU, thus supporting the reduction of health inequalities, including aspects of gender medicine. While focusing on promotion and prevention, this initiative should also support better knowledge and data, screening and early detection, diagnosis and treatment management, and patient quality of life. Another objective should be helping EU countries to transfer best practices, develop guidelines, and roll out innovative approaches, etc. This also means that the EU should name another European mission – to build healthcare systems that are more resilient to pandemics when it comes to cardio-vascular disease, in line with the efforts of the cancer mission, ultimately addressing the two NCDs with the highest burden on the European population. We also see a need to address other diseases, especially those which heavily impact European GDP – e.g. musculoskeletal conditions.

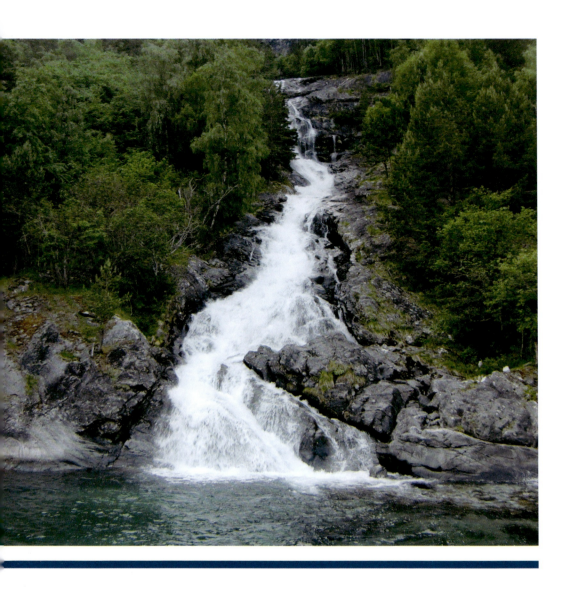

INT/962

**OPINION EUROPEAN ECONOMIC AND SOCIAL COMMITTEE
A PACT FOR RESEARCH AND INNOVATION IN EUROPE**

Paul Rübig, Panagiotis Gkofas (Co-Author)

1   Conclusions and recommendations

1.1   The EESC welcomes the fact that the Pact for Research and Innovation in Europe sets out commonly agreed values and principles for R&I and identifies, on a global, general level, the areas where Member States will jointly develop priority actions. The Pact thus supports the new European Research Area (ERA) while bearing in mind that research and innovation are largely national competences.

1.2   The Council recommendation is divided into major parts, which are addressed in the following sections:
1. Values and principles;
2. Priority areas for joint action;
3. Prioritising investments in R&D;
4. Policy coordination and monitoring and reporting.

1.3   In the future, Europe should make value creation, business and quality jobs out of Europe's R&D-results. One very important tool for making business, profit and jobs for Europe out of Europe's R&D-results is Intellectual Property Rights (IPR). The great importance of IPR and patents should be added to the paragraph on Value Creation and a clear IPR strategy for Europe should be developed in the framework of the Pact for the New ERA. This active and passive EU patent policy and patent strategy should be accompanied by an active and passive license strategy and a transparent monitoring system for the net global patent and license balance.

1.4   The EESC welcomes the Pact's clear call to deepen the ERA, i.e. to move from coordinating national policies to deeper integration of these policies, and its call to accelerate the twin green and digital transitions. Thus far, R&I in the EU 27 has still mainly been conducted in parallel working silos. These silos now have to be connected by massive "communication pipes", which the EESC believes must be one of the Pact's major objectives.

1.5   The EESC feels that, in view of the massive investments in Research, Technology, Innovation (RTI) in Asia (China, South Korea etc.), the EU has to substantially speed up its efforts in R&I, especially regarding the fast transformation of R&D results into innovative products and services, since Europe is lagging behind in this area, as clearly pointed out in COM(2020) 628.

1.6   The EESC would like to point out that R&I have to be speeded up in the EU and the digital transition achieved fast. A recently published EC report, the 2021 EU Industrial R&D Investment Scoreboard, shows that China has increased its R&D investments from 2020 to 2021 by 18.1%, the USA has increased its R&D investments from 2020 to 2021 by

9.1%, whereas the EU 27 have decreased their R&D investments by 2.2%. These transition processes have to be fair and just, not leaving behind any group of civil society, especially vulnerable citizens, European citizens living in remote regions or the social partners.

1.7 As pointed out in the new ERA, as well as in the Pact, the EU really needs a new vision, i.e. a New Deal for the EU's ERA. With just "more of the same" as its old RTI strategy, the EU will continue to fall behind the US and Asia (China, Korea, etc.) in R&I.

1.8 To date only a limited share of the EU population (the "usual suspects for R&I" only) have been engaged in the EU's R&I policies. However, modern socioeconomic research highlights the great importance of the Science-Technology-Society (STS) for strong performers in R&I. To contribute concretely with the objective of a stronger EU in the world, the EESC asks to include, in appropriate form, civil society organisations, social and economic partners (notably organisations representing MSMEs) at EU and national level in the European Commission's monitoring of the actions already deployed in 2022 by the new ERA Forum and related initiatives like the new European Citizens' Panels within the Conference on the Future of Europe. The so-called knowledge triangle (Higher Education, Basic and Applied Research, Commercialisation of new technology by Industry), which we are glad to see referenced in the Commission's Pact for R&I, too, is an important concept for boosting R&I. Within this concept of participation of EU civil society, it is important, too, to make sure that the workers on the shop floor – as well as vulnerable EU citizens – are included.

1.9 Within the new Pact for R&I Europe must prepare the soil for a more entrepreneurial culture such that risk-taking, innovative businesses are encouraged – MSMEs as well as start-ups. The well-known slogan "No risk, no fun" translates in innovation into "No risk, no new business, no new quality jobs".

1.10 There are many Commission documents and programmes on R&I. Thus, the EESC would appreciate the Commission clarifying the interlinkages between all its documents on R&I, including the Pact for R&I, the New Era, the European Missions, the EU Recovery and Resilience Plan and Horizon Europe in general.

1.11 Last but not least, the EESC wishes to point out that the EU's Pact for R&I and its new ERA should be designed and implemented in agreement with the United Nations' 17 Sustainable Development Goals (SDGs), which aim to achieve decent lives for all on a healthy planet by 2030.

2. General comments

2.1 The core Commission document, on which the Pact is based and to which the Pact refers, is COM(2020) 628 – A new ERA for Research and Innovation.

2.2 In March 2021, the EESC published an opinion[1] on A new ERA for Research and Innovation[2]. Many of the conclusions, recommendations and general comments contained in that EESC opinion are also valid for the Pact; some of them are reproduced in this document.

2.3 Bringing these R&I elements together in a single legal act will reaffirm Member States' political commitment to mobilise their R&I policies to tackle the challenges that Europe faces today, which are:

a) The twin transition (digital transition and green deal)

b) The post-pandemic recovery

c) The ever-fiercer global competition in RTI, especially from Asia (China, Korea, etc.).

All these challenges have to be tackled in a fair and just way, leaving no one behind, especially not vulnerable EU citizens.

2.4 Global RTI rankings and studies show that, in terms of global competition, the EU 27 are lagging behind the USA and Asia, especially China and Korea, where RTI is concerned, especially in terms of Key Enabling Technologies (KETs) (e.g. Artificial Intelligence, Machine Learning, Robotics, Digital Business Models, etc.). Challenges a) and b) are to be found in Commission communication COM(2021) 407. Challenge c) "global competition in RTI especially from Asia (China, Korea, etc.)" has been added intentionally by the EESC, because it feels that if the EU does not address this challenge successfully the EU will lose millions of qualified jobs to Asia and will thus lose wealth and quality of life for Europeans. RTI is the major generator of future quality jobs. If technological leadership in many industries moves to Asia, quality jobs will also move to Asia.

2.5 The European Research Council (ERC), too, has already issued an opinion on the Pact and the new ERA. The ERC, too, stresses very clearly that the EU is falling behind in comparison to Asia, especially China, regarding RTI, stating that "The pact for R&I may be the EU´s last chance to finally meet the goals of the original ERA to cement Europe's position as a leader in research and innovation"[3].

2.6 China has not only overtaken the EU regarding output in R&D and output in patents but, for around five years, has also very aggressively taken the global lead in setting technological

---

1   EESC opinion on A new European Research Area (ERA) for Research and Innovation, OJ C 220, 9.6.2021, p. 79.

2   COM(2020) 628.

3   Source: https://erc.europa.eu/news/pact-research-innovation-foundations-european-research-area-still-valid-and-

industry standards. For many decades, the US and Europe had monopolised the setting of industry standards. Setting the technology industry's standards has a very powerful role in global RTI, meaning that the nation that sets these standards has a competitive advantage. The EESC therefore strongly recommends that the Commission set out clear measures in the Pact, to uphold Europe's strong position in setting global technology industry standards.

2.7   The EESC feels that, in view of the massive investments in RTI in Asia (China, South Korea etc.), the EU has to substantially speed up its efforts in R&I, especially regarding the fast transformation of R&D results into innovative products and services. A recently published EC report, the 2021 EU Industrial R&D Investment Scoreboard, shows that China has increased its R&D investments from 2020 to 2021 by 18.1%, the USA has increased its R&D investments from 2020 to 2021 by 9.1%, whereas the EU 27 have decreased their R&D investments by 2.2%. The EU's measures to speed up R&I have to address multinationals headquartered in the EU, as well as MSMEs, since MSMEs, too, are threatened by competition from Asia and since most of the employment growth in Europe stems from MSMEs and start-ups, not from large enterprises.

2.8   The EESC welcomes the clear call made in the Pact for a deepening of the ERA, i.e. moving from the coordination of national policies to the deeper integration of these policies, as well as the call to accelerate the green and digital transition. Until now, R&I in the EU 27 has still mainly been conducted in parallel working silos. These silos now have to be connected by massive "communication pipes" which, in the EESC's view, must be one of the Pact's major objectives. Communication and cooperation are key driving forces for R&I.

2.9   As pointed out in the new ERA, as well as in the Pact, the EU really needs a new vision, i.e. a New Deal for the EU's ERA. With just 'more of the same' as its old RTI strategy, the EU will continue to fall behind the US and Asia (China, Korea, etc.) in R&I.

2.10   Many studies conclude, that knowledge transfer in R&I works primarily via heads, i.e. via job rotation between R&I organisations, as well as between EU Member States on a massive scale. The EESC recommends massively increasing knowledge transfer via heads, i.e. job rotations and researcher mobility programmes within the EU 27 on a huge scale. Knowledge transfer in R&I does not work via large documents: one cannot transfer the knowledge of five years' R&D work of any researcher by means of a 500-page R&D report.

2.11   The Pact refers to the ERA technology roadmaps. To the current knowledge of the EESC, an ERA roadmap for 2015-2020 is available, but the EESC is not aware of any ERA technology roadmap going beyond 2020. Technology strategies have to be planned for the long term, since a new technology does not happen overnight. Technology roadmaps need a lead time of at least 10 years. The EESC therefore encourages the

Commission to develop mid-term (2020-2030) and long-term (2020-2050) technology roadmaps following the publication of the new ERA.

2.12 The EESC welcomes the reference to the great importance of the so-called 'knowledge triangle' (Higher Education, Basic and Applied Research, Commercialisation of new tech by Industry)[4].

2.13 The EESC believes that, while it is true that research and (higher) education are key drivers of knowledge creation, they are not the key driver for innovation. Innovation – by definition – means the conversion of R&D results into innovative products and business. It is not the task of universities or of research institutes to develop innovative products and business. In this paragraph, enterprises, especially start-ups and entrepreneurs, are missing and their important role in the innovation process has to be added here. The European Innovation Council (EIC), the European Institute of Innovation and Technology Knowledge and Innovation Communities (EIT KIC) and other innovation schemes play an important role in this context.

2.14 According to the famous diagram of Professor Ansoff, only a small share of R&D projects (less than approx. 25%) eventually yield successful technical products on the market. Thus, one major focus within the EU's R&I pact and strategy has to be the effectiveness and efficiency of R&I. If, with intelligent means to ensure the effectiveness and efficiency of R&I, its rate of success can be increased from 25% to e.g. 28%, this would be an enormous success for Europe. The effectiveness and efficiency of R&I, while maintaining the EU's strong claim for excellence in research, could also substantially speed up Europe's R&I, which is desperately needed.

2.15 Regarding "Values and Principles", the EESC agrees that the values stated in this chapter are important, but to stop the EU falling behind the USA and Asia in the global R&I competition, additional principles are needed. It is stipulated the new ERA that the EU must speed up the conversion of R&D results into innovative products and services for the global markets. This urgently needed speeding-up requires, among other values and competences, entrepreneurship. Many global studies suggest that the EU is lagging behind substantially compared to the USA and Asia regarding entrepreneurship (e.g. regarding innovative digital business models).

2.16 Regarding "Value Creation", the EESC fully agrees on the very high importance of transforming 'knowledge' (i.e. R&D-results) into innovative, sustainable products and services. The pact

---

4   As highlighted in point 2(h) of the Proposal for a Council Recommendation (COM(2021) 407). Paragraph (h) reads: "Research and innovation and (higher) education are key drivers of innovation, knowledge creation, diffusion and use."

refers to the important role of basic research regarding generating breakthrough discoveries and knowledge. However, creating 'value for Europe' needs more than generating breakthrough discoveries: There are – unfortunately – numerous examples in which European researchers have been generating breakthrough discoveries, but entrepreneurs and innovative companies from USA and Asia have been making business and profit out of Europe's R&D results and the jobs went from Europe to USA and Asia. Europe should not let happen this again.

2.17 Europe should in the future make value, business and quality jobs out of Europe's own R&D-results. One very important tool for making business, profit and jobs for Europe out of Europe's R&D-results is patents. The great importance of IPR (Intellectual Property Rights) should be added to the paragraph on Value Creation and a clear IPR strategy for Europe should be developed in the framework of the Pact for the new ERA. This active and passive EU patent policy and patent strategy should be accompanied by an active and passive license strategy and a transparent monitoring system for the net global patent and license balance.

2.18 In point 2 of the Proposal for a Council Recommendation[5], the priority areas for the EU's R&I are given. The following priority areas for R&I topics are also given in COM(2020) 628:
- Artificial intelligence
- Microelectronics
- Quantum Computing
- 5G
- Renewable energy
- Hydrogen technologies
- Zero emission and smart mobility

2.19 The EESC wishes to reiterate that, while it agrees that these seven priority areas[6] are very important, the following key technologies and sectors should be added:
- Space technologies;
- Clean water and sanitation,
- New, high-tech materials with high future potential for the EU, e.g. Graphene
- Technologies for manufacturing goods and food;
- The clinical research, pharmaceutical and bio-technological sectors;
- Digital business models in general;
- Technologies (hardware and software) for emergency preparedness (blackouts, disruption of digital communications e.g. by cyber crime etc.).

---

5   COM(2021) 407
6   As given in COM(2020) 628.

2.20   The EU 27 – unfortunately – have a significant brain drain of excellent researchers to the USA and increasingly to Asia, too. This brain drain has to be stopped and should be converted into a brain gain. Among others, the following principles are very important for an excellent, globally leading, fast RTI performance:

- Recognition and fair remuneration of excellent researchers in the EU 27, in particular excellent female researchers (see poor gender balance in RTI in the EU 27).
- Efficient Communication, Collaboration and Cooperation (the three important "Cs" of innovation!)
- Increasing EU and national funding for research centres and universities, based on competitive bidding processes, thus insuring that the 'best-of-the-best' researchers get the money (not funding by a 'watering can' to all research centres).

2.21   One major goal of the EU's new ERA is value creation. Thus, the EESC feels that the paragraph "Knowledge Valorisation" is very important. In this paragraph, the importance of cooperation and interlinkages between all R&I actors is highlighted. This is important, but **not** enough for 'Knowledge Valorisation'.

2.22   Issues that are equally important for value creation for Europe are:

- a commitment to rapid conversion of R&D results into innovative products, services and ultimately into values, business and quality jobs. This requires, inter alia, a much more entrepreneurial culture in Europe as well as a positive attitude to taking risks: fast launch of innovative products always incurs risks too.
  The well-known slogan "No risk, no fun" translates innovation into "No risk, no business, no new jobs";
- a clear technology roadmap, especially regarding KETs and FETs (Key Enabling Technologies);
- a clear IPR strategy for the new ERA.

2.23   Regarding "Deepening a truly functioning internal market for knowledge", knowledge – without any doubt – is very important, since the 21st century is the century of knowledge. However, it is also very important to give a new boost to production of all hardware in Europe. 20 years ago, the EU thought that the production of goods could be moved to Asia, while keeping production-related R&D in Europe. This turned out to be a mistake. R&D always follows production, sooner or later. Thus, to bring back at least a portion of production and its related jobs from Asia to Europe, the EU needs to make great efforts. This would also go a long way towards solving the problem of unemployment, which is a particularly big problem in some countries in Southern Europe.

2.24   A lesson which Europe, too, has learned from the corona pandemic: The production of almost all basic medications and vaccines has moved from Europe to Asia in the last 20 or 30 years. Europe has lost its sovereignty in many important products and medicines. Microchips are another example where European industry, especially the car industry, is suffering massively at the moment. Other examples where Europe – unfortunately – is almost fully dependent on Asia are batteries for electric vehicles, hydrogen technologies. (While European car producers still are experimenting with prototypes of hydrogen powered cars, Toyota, Honda and Hyundai already mass produce them and sell them regularly). Asia also is by far the leader in optical technologies, 5G communication technologies, artificial intelligence, machine learning, robotics and many others KETs and FETs (Key Enabling and Future Technologies). In the Pact for R&I Europe must make regaining sovereignty in key technologies a clear priority.

2.25   Europe is on the one hand facing the challenge of high unemployment among young people, especially in some countries in Southern Europe and, on the other, the challenge of a shortage of highly qualified STEM (Science, Technology, Engineering, Mathematics) graduates, especially a severe shortage of engineers in all fields of ICT and digitalisation, e-mobility and in technologies for renewable energies. It is often forgotten that it is primarily engineers that convert R&D results achieved by researchers into technical products. Due to demographic changes (our ageing society) and due to the fact that most countries in Europe are failing to attract more women students to engineering studies, this problem will increase in the near future. Of course, measures to attract more women students to engineering studies have to be increased in the EU on a huge scale. In addition, smart programmes for attracting highly-qualified engineers from non-EU Member States have to be generated by the Pact for R&I. The global RTI-competition will increasingly become a global talent war, and up to now, the EU has performed badly in this global talent war for talents compared to the US, for example.

2.26   Last but not least, the EESC wishes to point out that EU's Pact for R&I and its new ERA should be designed and implemented in agreement with the United Nations' 17 Sustainable Development Goals, which aim to achieve decent lives for all on a healthy planet by 2030.

UNITED NATIONS SUSTAINABLE DEVELOPMENT GOALS 2, 6, 7, 14

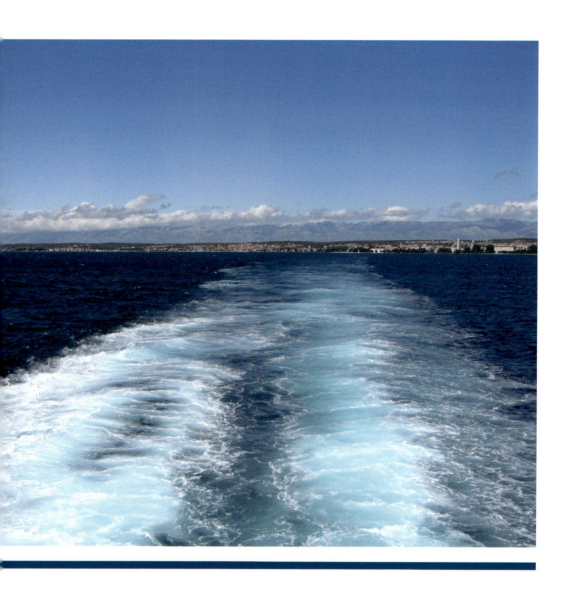

WATER AND SUSTAINABLE AGRIFOOD SYSTEMS

Antonia María Lorenzo López
(BIOAZUL SL, University of Córdoba – WEARE Research Group),
Rafael Casielles Restoy (BIOAZUL SL)

INTRODUCTION

Food sustainability and security are among the main global challenges in the current context of climate change the effects of which are widely threatening the whole food value chain worldwide, from production to consumption.

There are several definitions of Sustainable Food Systems (SFS) proposed by recognised organisations and scientists. For the purpose of this report, the one proposed by FAO is being used (1):

*A **sustainable food system (SFS)** is a food system that delivers food security and nutrition for all in such a way that the economic, social, and environmental bases to generate food security and nutrition for future generations are not compromised. This means that:*
- *It is profitable throughout (**economic sustainability**);*
- *It has broad-based benefits for society (**social sustainability**); and*
- *It has a positive or neutral impact on the natural environment (**environmental sustainability**).*

In addition, the definition provided by the Science Advice for Policy By European Academies in the report "A sustainable food system for the European Union" issued in 2020 (2) clearly states the needed global approach to be considered when proposing different transformation measures to turn current food systems more sustainable and just.

"Provides and promote safe, nutritious, and healthy food of low environmental impact for all current and future EU citizens in a manner that itself also protects and restores the natural environment and its ecosystem services, is robust and resilient, economically dynamic, just and fair, and socially acceptable and inclusive. It does so without compromising the availability of nutritious and healthy food for people living outside the EU, nor impairing their natural environment."

But the transition from current food systems, based on linear economy models which are no longer viable, towards more circular and sustainable models is quite a challenging task.

Therefore, actions should be taken at global level to address the diversity of the food systems in a multidisciplinary approach involving all key value chain actors to ensure the provision of food for a growing population with increasingly limited resources, including water, in a context of climate change.

Examples of initiatives at global level promoting a food system shift are the European Food Forum , the EU Carbon+ Farming Coalition, EU Green Deal's Farm to Fork Strategy, Circular Economy Strategies, and the United Nations' Sustainable Development Goals (SDGs), among others.

AGRIFOOD SYSTEMS MAIN CHALLENGES

There are relevant barriers to overcome the transition challenges of current agri-food systems that evidence that this transition is not possible to happen in a business-as-usual linear manner.

Ensuring food for all in the coming decades of a growing population, 10 billion projected by 2050, will demand **50% more food by 2050** (3) if there are no rapid changes in the **consumption patterns** and levels of **food waste generated**.

It is estimated that around one third of the total food produced is lost or wasted across all stages of the food supply chains (4,5). In terms of water, the food not being eaten accounts for 25% of the world´s fresh water supply (6).

Climate change is putting global food production at risk by limiting natural resources, including water availability and quality, the degradation of ecosystems, arable land and soils, and the loss of biodiversity.

Moreover, the effects of climate change in rural areas, together with the lack of services such as digital connection, are forcing people to move to cities, with a foreseen 66% of world population living in urban areas by 2050. This is causing the depopulation of rural areas and thus limiting the labour force for agriculture.

With regards specifically to water, the current scarcity and the more frequent droughts are becoming an issue of growing concern worldwide. They are affecting more and more regions across the globe, even traditionally wet ones, and represent a major challenge for our society. Far from diminishing, the impact of water scarcity and droughts will worsen in the coming years mainly as a result of climate change.

Figure 1 shows the map of the water stress as the ratio of total water withdrawals to available renewable surface and groundwater supplies.

It is foreseen that by 2020 more than half of the world population will live in water stress areas. (7). The agrifood industry is characterised by being water intensive, accounting for 70% of the total water withdrawals on average and by generating large amounts of waste and wastewater. The food and land use systems account for 92% of the global water foot-print (8).

At the same time, according to Kala Vairavamoorthy, the Executive Director of IWA "85% of the global wastewater is not being treated" (9). As shown in figure 2a, large amounts of wastewater are still not being treated that could be discharged to water bodies causing enviromental problems such as eutrofication (figure 2b).

Moreover, in the current context of climate variability, enormous difficulties in forecasting and estimating water resources in the immediate future implies the use of non-conventional resources such as reclaimed water is of increasing interest. Despite the potential of reclaimed water, which is estimated at 6,000 Mm3 by the European Commission, there are still barriers for wider implementation.

Therefore, it is crucial not only to consider in the hydrological planning the infrastructures needed to treat the wastewater, but also to consider non-conventional water sources, such as the reclaimed water, as a complementary source whose use will support the preservation and restauration of

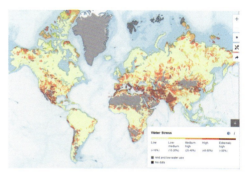

Figure 1: Global water stress map

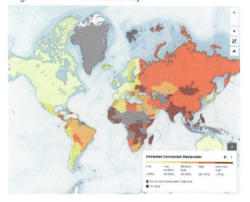

Figure 2a: Global untreated connect wastewater map

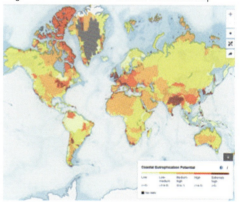

Figure 2b: Global coastal eutrophication potential map
(source 1-2b: www.wri.org/applications/aqueduct/water-risk-atlas)

conventional surface and ground water sources. According to the Water and Circular Economy working group of the Conama Foundation report "Agua y Economia Circular", the hydrological planning is analogous to the eco-design in the frame of the circular economy approach (10).

The transversal measures to be implemented in the water planning and management should be adapted to the climate change scenario and include all water uses (industrial, urban, and agricultural) and users and should be focused on decreasing the consumption and increasing the efficiency. This is the only pathway for a sustainable development, especially for agrifood systems which are the backbone of our economy and essential to fulfil the 2030 Agenda and the Paris Agreement on Climate Change.

Adaptation and mitigation solutions are therefore needed to manage and use water in the best possible way and to recover resources from water effluents as secondary raw materials, formerly considered as residues/waste.

RECLAIMED WATER USE IN AGRICULTURE

Reclaimed water is treated wastewater that meets discharge parameters and subsequently undergoes additional treatment in order to meet the quality standards required for a specific use according to the legal framework of application.

Reclaimed water usage, a **well-recognised measure for climate change adaptation**, gives circularity to the water resource and also potentiality to the embedded valuable compounds, such as crop nutrients, contributing to the preservation of natural resources and natural capital.

The use of reclaimed water accounts for many advantages:
- Availability of a constant source of water independent of climate events.
- Incentives to extend wastewater treatment.
- Supply of water and nutrients (fertiliser savings), thus enabling irrigators to cut costs by reducing fertiliser consumption.
- Reduction of diffuse pollution, eutrophication as crops absorb the nutrients in the reclaimed water that do not accumulate in water bodies.
- Net increase of water resources in coastal areas.
- Lower impacts and costs than other alternative water resources (e.g. desalinated water or water transfers).

In addition, the use of reclaimed water contributes to the achievement of the UN2030 Agenda, as it is aligned to the SGD6 and SGD12 targets, such as:

6.3 By 2030, improve water quality by reducing pollution, eliminating dumping and minimising release of hazardous chemicals and materials, halving the proportion of untreated wastewater and substantially increasing recycling and safe reuse globally.

6.4 By 2030, substantially increase water-use efficiency across all sectors and ensure sustainable withdrawals and supply of freshwater to address water scarcity and substantially reduce the number of people suffering from water scarcity.

6.5 By 2030, implement integrated water resources management at all levels, including through transboundary cooperation as appropriate.

6.A By 2030, expand international cooperation and capacity-building support to developing countries in water- and sanitation-related activities and programmes, including water harvesting, desalination, water efficiency, wastewater treatment, recycling and reuse technologies.

6.6 By 2020, protect and restore water-related ecosystems, including mountains, forests, wetlands, rivers, aquifers, and lakes.

12.1 Implement the 10-year framework of programmes on sustainable consumption and production, all countries taking action, with developed countries taking the lead, taking into account the development and capabilities of developing countries.

12.2 By 2030, achieve the sustainable management and efficient use of natural resources.

12.4 By 2020, achieve the environmentally sound management of chemicals and all wastes throughout their life cycle, in accordance with agreed international frameworks, and significantly reduce their release to air, water, and soil in order to minimise their adverse impacts on human health and the environment.

12.5 By 2030, substantially reduce waste generation through prevention, reduction, recycling, and reuse.

12.8 By 2030, ensure that people everywhere have the relevant information and awareness for sustainable development and lifestyles in harmony with nature.

But the implementation of large water reuse projects to harvesting the enormous potential of reclaimed water for agriculture, also faces significant barriers such as:

- It requires adequate infrastructure for the treatment of the wastewater and pipping network.
- An analytical monitoring plan is needed to ensure quality at different points of compliance, fulfilling the applicable legal framework.
- There is still an unrealistic perception of risks associated to the use of reclaimed water, which causes some social reluctance about its use by farmers, which prolongs this situation and makes agricultural activity increasingly unsustainable.

In addition, there is a lack of awareness and recognition of the extent of the water scarcity we face. Many aquifers are strongly affected by salinisation and falling water table levels, which means that obtaining water is increasingly expensive and the water is of poorer quality.

Successful case studies and technical and scientific evidence is needed to promote the use of the reclaimed water in agriculture, to leverage the investment for infrastructures and to overcome current reluctancy, thus highly impacting water governance and management.

RICHWATER PROJECT CASE STUDY

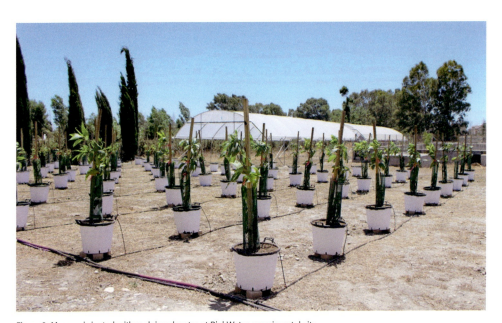

Figure 3: Mangos irrigated with reclaimed water at RichWater experimental site

RichWater is an innovation action funded by Horizon 2020 which tested and validated an integrated solution for water reuse in agriculture. A system prototype with the capacity of treatment for 150 m³/day was demonstrated for the treatment and reclamation of municipal wastewater of the town of Algarrobo within the region of La Axarquia (Malaga, Spain). This region is located on the southern coast of Spain. It combines rural areas in the interior with strong agricultural activity and densely populated coastal areas with high affluence of tourists during the summer. Indeed, La Axarquia is the main producer of sub-tropical crops in Europe. The region suffers from water scarcity with the overexploitation of groundwater, low levels of water reservoirs, and is at risk of desertification. Wastewater is directly flowing into the Mediterranean Sea, together with high N & P leaching from agriculture, causing eutrophication at the coastal zone and losses of valuable water resources which are discharged while the region is running out of water. Approximately 40% of river waters are at certain risk of non-compliance with the EU's Water Framework Directive (WFD). Due to the need for irrigation and intensive fertiliser application, local agriculture is highly vulnerable to climate change effects. Therefore, the local government started in 2021 with an upgrade of existing infrastructure in local WWTPs to make reclaimed water available to farmers for irrigation. To control nutrient supply from wastewater and to overcome farmers' reluctance on using reclaimed wastewater, adequate strategies need to be defined; this will also avoid pollution increases in water bodies.

The RichWater system includes an MBR and an integrated irrigation system with a mixing station. The MBR was designed to keep nutrients, while pathogens and other pollutants are removed. This leads to a nutrient-rich effluent adequate for use in food crops irrigation. The MBR has been verified under the Environmental Technology Verification (ETV) programme supported by the European Commission. The verified MBR guarantees a high quality of the effluent complying with the legal standards for water reuse set in the EU regulation 2020/741. The ETV verification has been very important to overcome end-users' reluctance. Thus, farmers gained confidence in the quality of the water due to the "quality label" provided by the ETV verification, which was conducted by an external verification body.

	BOD5 (mg O$_2$/l)	COD (mg O$_2$/l)	TS (mg/l)	TN (mg N/l)	TP (mg/l)	TK (mg/l)	Turbidity (NTU)
Min	93.00	239.00	106.00	25.00	3.30	8.80	2.60
Max	232.00	646.00	397.00	67.00	12.00	25.00	349.00
Average	163.25	408.31	210.06	38.81	5.97	14.81	120.48
Min	<15	15.00	< 8	16.00	0.16	8.10	0.16
Max	<15	32.00	< 8	45.00	12.00	24.00	2.30
Average	<15	23.67	< 8	26.00	4.34	14.43	0.69
Removal %	90.81%	94.20%	96.19%	33.01%	27.31%	2.62%	99.43%

Table 1: RichWater performance parameters verified through ETV

Absence of E. Coli, legionella, and salmonella

On the other hand, the irrigation system counts with a nutrient monitoring tool to optimise fertilisation and to avoid the over-fertilisation of crops irrigated with reclaimed water. The RichWater system was specifically designed for the reuse of the effluent in agriculture. The mixing station mixes the appropriate proportion of freshwater and the treated wastewater coming from the MBR, which is then fed into the fertigation module (drip irrigation). The appropriate mixing level is determined by monitoring the level of nutrient content in the soil via sensors. Thus, the nutrients contained in the wastewater (mainly nitrogen, phosphorus, and potassium) remain after the treatment whilst pathogens are removed. These nutrients are directly assimilable by crops and therefore implies the important saving of ferstilisers for farmers. In this sense, RichWater is able to recover 72% of N and 63% of P from the reclaimed water (11).

REFERENCES

1. Nguyen, H. (2018) 'Sustainable food systems Concept and framework', FAO. Available at: https://www.fao.org/3/ca2079en/CA2079EN.pdf.
2. SAPEA, (2020) 'A sustainable food system for the European Union', Berlin: SAPEA. Available at: https://www.sapea.info/wp-content/uploads/sustainable-food-system-report.pdf.
3. Addams, L., *et al.* (2022) 'Charting Our Water Future Economic frameworks to inform decision-making', 2030 Water Resources Group. Available at: https://www.mckinsey.com/~/media/mckinsey/dotcom/client_service/sustainability/pdfs/charting%20our%20water%20future/charting_our_water_future_full_report_.ashx.
4. FAO (2013) 'Food Wastage Footprint: Impacts on Natural Resources', Rome: FAO. Available at: https://reliefweb.int/report/world/food-wastage-footprint-impacts-natural-resources.
5. // Shukla, P.R., *et al.* (2019) 'Summary for Policymakers'. In: *Climate Change and Land: an IPCC special report on climate change, desertification, land degradation, sustainable land management, food security, and greenhouse gas fluxes in terrestrial ecosystems'*, IPCC. Available at: https://www.ipcc.ch/site/assets/uploads/sites/4/2020/02/SPM_Updated-Jan20.pdf
6. Hall, K., Guo, J., Dore, M., Chow, C. (2009) 'The Progressive Increase of Food Waste in America and Its Environmental Impact', PloS ONE 4(11): e790. https://doi.org/10.1371/journal.pone.0007940
7. UN-Water (2020) 'United Nations World Water Development Report 2020: Water and Climate Change', Paris: UNESCO. Available at: https://unesdoc.unesco.org/ark:/48223/pf0000372985.locale=en
8. World Economic Forum (2022) 'Transforming Food Systems with Farmers: A Pathway for the EU', The World Economic Forum. Available at: https://www3.weforum.org/docs/WEF_Transforming_Food_Systems_with_Farmers_A_Pathway_for_the_EU_2022.pdf
9. Vairavamoorthy, K. (2019),'The challanges of the water sector', *SIGA International Water Conference*. Available at: https://www.youtube.com/watch?v=s6fhdqKSrxM&list=PL6CTjn4hdBFdPULdpUUFU4ucnEO6N_NW7
10. Van Hove, E., *et al.* (2019) 'Agua y Economía Circular', Fundación Conama. Available at: http://www.fundacionconama.org/wp-content/uploads/2019/09/Agua-y-Econom%C3%ADa-Circular.pdf
11. Muñoz-Sánchez, D., *et al.* (2018) 'Assessing Quality of Reclaimed Urban Wastewater from Algarrobo Municipality to Be Used for Irrigation', *Journal of Water Resource and Protection*, 10, 1090-1105. https://doi.org/10.4236/jwarp.2018.1011064

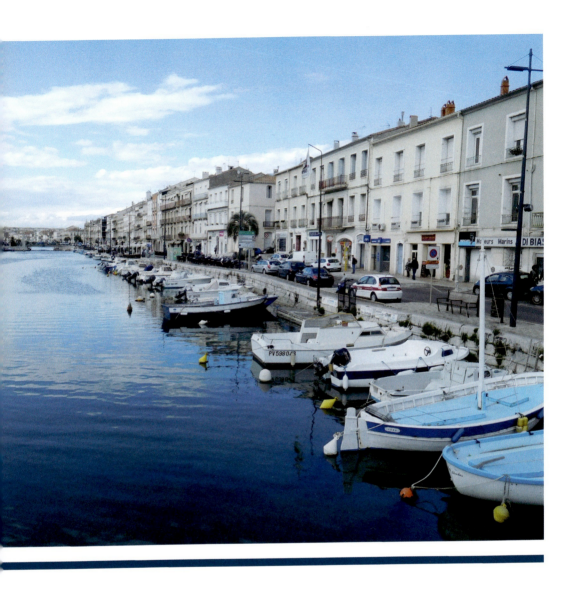

WATER EUROPE'S VISION FOR A WATER-SMART SOCIETY

Durk Krol (Executive Director of Water Europe)

Since Water Europe first published its vision for a Water-Smart Society in 2016, its concepts have found wide recognition in the water-related research, innovation, and policy debate in Europe and beyond. At the beginning of 2023, a new edition will be launched, laying out a sharper, better defined and fine-tuned policy-oriented vision based on the latest developments and data, progressive insights in Water Europe's goals and strategies, and building on the experience of having worked with the current edition for six years now. It is my great pleasure to provide a preview of the new vision in this important book on achieving the SDG6.

The vision for a Water-Smart Society aims to set out the pathways towards better use, valorisation, and stewardship of our water resources by society and businesses while developing resilient and sustainable solutions for our key global water challenges. It describes how these challenges can be turned into opportunities to develop new technologies, solutions, businesses, and governance models for the Water-Smart Society of the future. This vision imagines a future of full water security, safety, resilience, and sustainability for all societal functions, while protecting our environment: all relevant stakeholders are involved in the sustainable governance of our inclusive water system, in a way that meets present ecological, social, and economic needs without compromising the ability to meet those needs in the future; water scarcity as well as pollution of ground and surface water are avoided while biodiversity is being restored; water, energy and resource loops are largely closed to foster a circular economy; the water system is resilient and robust against climate change events and water-dependent businesses thrive as a result of forward-looking research and innovation.

A WATER-SMART SOCIETY IS DEFINED AS:

A society in which the true value of water is recognised and realised, and all available water sources are managed in such a way that water scarcity and pollution is avoided; the water system is resilient against droughts and floods which are exacerbated by climate change, and all relevant stakeholders are engaged to guarantee sustainable water governance, while water and resource loops are largely closed to foster a circular economy.

THE MODEL FOR A WATER-SMART SOCIETY

The **Water Europe model for a Water-Smart Society** involves one core value, three key objectives, and five innovation concepts to drive the development of essential solutions but more importantly to bring RTD results to market and achieve systemic innovation to our water system.

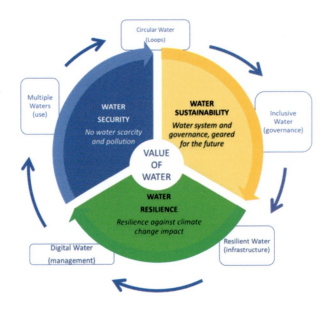

Water Europe Water-Smart Society Model

One core-value

The Value of Water – an essential concept at the core of Water Europe's vision for a *Water-Smart Society*, expressing water as a human right as well as the importance of water for our society at large, including enabling all our economic activities, societal functions related to health and well-being for all citizens regardless of their ability to pay, as well as the (potential) economic value that can be accomplished by valorising dissolved raw materials and the kinetic and thermal energy of water systems offering a unique sustainable source serving a circular economy.

Three core-objectives

Water Security: core-objective of the Water-Smart Society, to safeguard sustainable *access to enough affordable and healthy water as well as ecosystems* for sustaining good health and socio-economic development and for ensuring protection against water-related disasters such as the consequences of climate change.

Water Sustainability: core-objective of the Water-Smart Society ensuring water infrastructure, as well as management and use that is *economically and environmentally sustainable* in a way that meets present ecological, social, and economic needs without compromising the ability to meet those needs in the future.

Water Resilience: core-objective of the Water-Smart Society securing *long-term resilience* in which our natural and anthropogenic water systems can withstand unexpected disruptive events and prevent serious consequences such as droughts and floods while guaranteeing the reliability of the water system.

5 Innovation concepts

Circular water – important concept underpinning the Water Europe vision for a Water-Smart Society, outlining a critical element of the sustainable and circular water system of the future that *minimises water losses and fosters a resilient and water secure system.*

Inclusive water – an important concept underlying Water Europe's vision, defining *a water system whose governance reflects in a balanced way the interests of all stakeholders* in designing, managing, and maintaining a secure, resilient, and sustainable Water-Smart Society.

Resilient water – key concept underpinning the Water Europe vision for a Water-Smart Society, which focuses on a *resilient and reliable hybrid grey and green water system*, designed to withstand severe external and internal shocks without compromising the essential functions, including dealing with floods and droughts due to climate change. **Multiple-waters** – important concept underlying the Water Europe vision in which *multiple water sources and qualities (fresh groundwater and surface water, rainwater, brackish water, brine, grey water, black water, recycled water)* are part of a water-secure, resilient, and sustainable water system as a solid fundamental aspect of a Water-Smart Society.

Digital water – important concept underpinning the Water Europe vision based on a world where all people, devices, and processes are connected through the "Internet of Everything," leading to capillary networks capable of monitoring the *water system* from the producers all the way down to the individual user, as such generating continuous flows of valuable data (big data) for innovative Decision Support systems at different governance levels.

BUILDING A WATER-SMART SOCIETY

Water Europe envisions a significantly transformed water sector with respect to the current state of play. The innovation concepts defined above as well as measurable targets towards water security, sustainability, and resilience will drive decision-makers towards this transition and new water-smart economics. The transition to a Water-Smart Society will be enabled by new technologies and their combinations, created within inclusive open innovation environments, such as Water-Oriented Living Labs[1] and a redesigned water infrastructure.

Water-Oriented Living Labs are relevant innovation ecosystems that promote the co-creation, testing, and evaluation of innovations in representative real-life environments with the aim of realising a 'Water-Smart Society.' They are very important for the innovation process leading towards a Water-Smart Society. It takes research and development out of laboratories and sets it in real-life contexts. This allows for a better understanding of what triggers innovations and of those innovations that prove to be successful in different environmental, social, and cultural contexts. A Living Lab is not only a network of infrastructures and services but also a collaborative ecosystem that has been established to sustain community-driven innovations in a multi-stakeholder context.

Water Europe (WE) is the recognised voice for and promotor of water-related innovation and RTD in Europe. It is a purpose-driven multi-stakeholder association with over 250 members representing the whole diversity of the innovative water eco-system, including industry, research, water-service providers, technology suppliers, and public authorities. WE was initiated in 2004 by the European Union as a European Technology Platform.

---

1   Water-Oriented Living Labs Notebook Series: Water-Oriented Living Lab Notebook Series #2. Definitions, practices, and assessment methods.

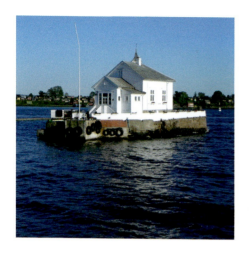
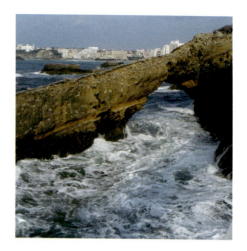
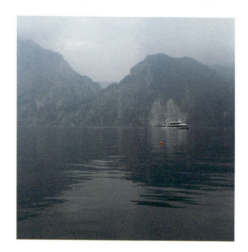
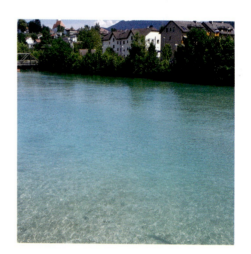
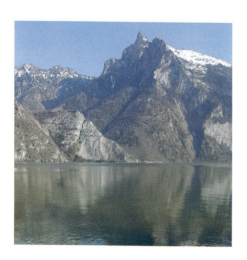
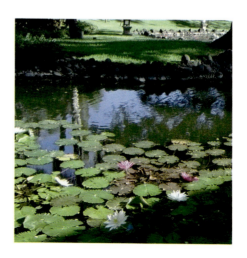

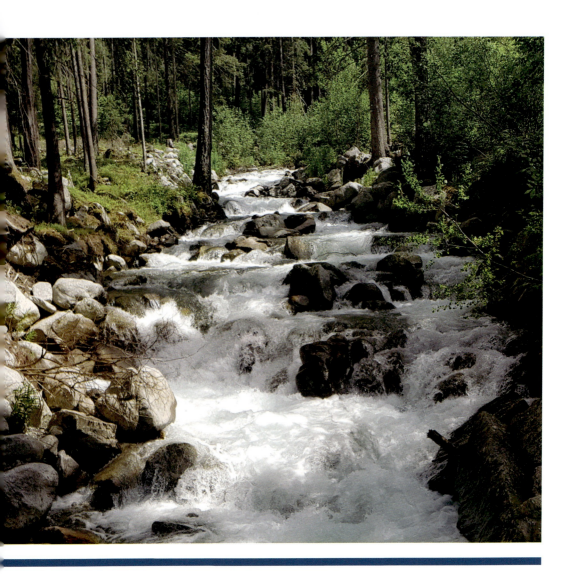

SDG6 – WATER IS A HUMAN RIGHT
(UN GENERAL ASSEMBLY 2010)

Johannes Pfaffenhuemer (Founder of Water of Life GmbH)

WATER OF LIFE - HEALTH CARE FROM THE SOURCE TO THE TABLE!

"Living water – source of health – water is life – water heals!"

Summary: Our health, the key to happiness in life!

Health is a state of complete physical, mental, and social well-being / WHO 1986 Ottawa Charter. "Health is not everything, but without health everything is nothing – nine tenths of our happiness are based on health alone, with it everything becomes a source of enjoyment!" wrote the philosopher Arthur Schopenauer (1788–1860).

Water scientists understand **"living water"** to mean natural, pure deep water that comes to the surface as a mature artesian spring of its own accord. It is quality water with high cell availability. (1) Water plays an increasingly important role as a **"fountain of youth"** in medicine, as confirmed by new studies and current scientific findings.

BACKGROUND - WATER AS A SOURCE OF HEALTH, DEVELOPMENT, AND SUSTAINABILITY

The global situation for quality drinking water is as follows:
– Up to 2.2 billion people worldwide have no access to clean drinking water
– 4.2 billion people suffer from inadequate sanitary and hygienic living conditions (drinking water pipes, sewage system)
– 40% of all schools worldwide have no toilets
– 1 in 3 people worldwide do not have the opportunity to wash their hands at home
– 700 million people could be forced to leave their homes by 2030 due to a lack of water
– Expected increase in demand for water by 2050: 55%
– 50% of all hospital beds worldwide are occupied by patients as a result of unclean water
– Virtual water is the total amount of fresh water used in the production of something. For example, about 140 litres of water are needed to produce a cup of coffee – especially when cultivating the necessary amount of coffee beans. 7,500 litres of fresh water are needed for a T-shirt, 20,000 litres for 1 laptop, 27,000 litres for 1 kg of beef, and around 400,000 litres for a car.
– **Sources: Federal Ministry for Economic Cooperation and Development in Germany, UN study from 2016**

WATER IS LIFE

Water is life and it is impossible to imagine our everyday life without it. Every day we drink, wash, cook, and water our flowers, meadows, and fields. We go to the pool, shower, and take a full bath. We are fortunate to have enough fresh water available, and unfortunately, we often forget that clean water is not a given in most parts of the world.

SPRING WATER AS THE ELIXIR OF LIFE

The best water for the human organism is natural, living, spring water that is low in minerals. Water transports absorbed nutrients, eliminates metabolic waste products, and maintains the osmotic pressure of the cells. This makes it the most important food for humans. Our bodily water content changes with age: Newborns have a water content of up to 85%, adults have a water content of approx. 65% – due to the physique, the water content in women is approx. 5-10% less than in men. With age, the proportion of water in both sexes falls below 50%, meaning that older people are more at risk of dehydration.

LIVING WATER FROM ARTESIAN SPRINGS

Artesian wells are springs of water that flow from deep within the Earth towards the surface via their own natural pressure. If the water emerges from a natural opening, it is called an artesian spring – named after the Artois region in northern France (since 1126). Since time immemorial, these springs have been referred to as "Holy Bründl (fountains)" throughout the Alps. Because of this natural process, the molecular structure of the water is preserved. The long-term flow of the water through rock strata keeps it pure and free of toxins. It is enriched with minerals and energies and thus carries a lot of information from the Earth's interior to the surface. One also speaks of mature water, which also has a special crystalline structure.

EPIGENETICS AND THE IMPORTANCE OF LIVING WATER

"Perhaps the mother of the cell was a water droplet," suggests Dr. Noemi Kempe, physicist from Moscow and head of the Institute for Biosensors and Bioenergetic Environmental Research (IBBU) in Graz/Austria. Cells are the elementary particles of all living things. Epigenetics deals with hereditary changes in gene regulation without directly changing the DNA sequence. Epigenetic changes can be initiated by chemical or physical environmental factors, but biological, psychological, and social factors are also able to model the epigenome. "We have unprecedented power over our genes and those of our children," says Dr. Kempe, because "heredity is the passing on of information to the next generation." And "we can change the epigenome with consciousness!" Water plays a decisive role in all processes in living material. Thus, the cell mass is 70% water, and it keeps its shape because water in liquid form is practically incompressible. Water has a transport function and is fully integrated into all information processes. "It is totally necessary to be careful about how much and what water you drink," recommends Dr. Kempe. (3)

THE PROBLEM WITH FREE RADICALS

A lack of water makes us age earlier. Dehydrated cells that are deprived of fluid break down mitochondria. The loss of cell water causes cells to shrink faster, making them more susceptible to attack by free radicals, bacteria, and viruses. Every day we are exposed to free radicals. The main sources of damage are environmental pollution, smoking or passive smoking, stress (including physical exertion such as sport), and radiation (X-rays, cosmic rays, air travel). Free radicals are molecules that become unstable as soon as they lose an electron. In order to regain their stability, these molecules quickly react with other compounds and try to grab the needed electron. The attacked molecule loses its electron, becoming a free radical itself and stealing an electron from the neighbouring molecule, triggering a chain reaction. As we age, our cell protection decreases due to a lack of antioxidant enzymes.

YOUR BODY IS NOT SICK, IT IS THIRSTY!

Dehydration is the root cause of many chronic diseases. This is what Dr. F. Batmanghelidj M.D. said in 2003 in his lecture on the healing power of water – held at "The Governmental Health Forum" in Washington, D.C., USA. He points out that as many people as possible should know the following truths about water:

- Earth and man are one: 71% of the Earth's surface is covered with water. Our body also consists largely of water, on average 70%.
- Many "diseases" are caused by dehydration
- Water regulates most functions of the body
- Water is necessary to avoid stress
- Dehydration and lack of salt cause high blood pressure
- Knowledge of the benefits of water is an educational subject

"The brain is made up of more than 90% water. The eyes are the sensory organs with the most water. The water transports vibrations that we send out and also receives them again." Prof. Gerald Pollok, a water researcher at the University of Washington, discovered the fourth aggregate form, the 4th dimension of water. Water organises at hydrophilic (wettable) interfaces. Links to the work of Dr. Gerald Pollok can be found at www.waterjournal.org

Lack of water as a cause of headaches and migraines: According to the German Migraine and Headache Society (DMKG), in Germany alone at least 3 million people suffer from headaches every day and 10 million have migraines regularly. Recent studies by British neurologist Dr. Joseph N. Blau show that dehydration often triggers both headaches and migraines.

Living water reduces cellulite: Cellulite is an accumulation of metabolic waste products in the connective tissue. Body waste is caused by drug residues, dental toxins, toxins, environmental toxins, food, animal proteins, refined carbohydrates, sugar, and many more causes. These metabolic waste products cause hyperacidity and unsightly dents on the buttocks, thighs, and upper arms. Cellulite is always caused by over-acidification of the body. Successful deacidification of the body is possible in many ways.

In addition to exercise in the fresh air, massages, and alkaline baths, mindful eating habits are helpful:
1. **Avoiding acid-forming foods:** alcohol, coffee, cola, etc.
2. **Increasing the proportion of alkaline-forming foods:** fruit, vegetables, salads – these foods also consist 70% of pure water.
3. **Flushing out the stored metabolic waste products with 3-5 litres of living, pure, healthy water** (depending on body weight). Living water has the power of artesian water and has the best conditions that the cells need to release the toxins in the body as quickly as possible. "Dead water stores up, living water washes out!" (Johann Abfalter)

Living water prevents obesity: "Drinking water should be a compulsory subject in schools," says Dr. Mathilde Kersting from the Research Institute for Child Nutrition (FKE): "Children have a water deficit!" This is demonstrably measurable in urine samples. Children who drink enough water can concentrate better and have a 31% lower risk of becoming overweight.

LIVING WATER, OUR "FOUNTAIN OF YOUTH" - IT KEEPS OUR CELLS YOUNG

Nowhere else can you see the age of someone as quickly as in the skin – if the body cells are fit and young, this is particularly evident in the face. Why is the aging process so different? The answer lies in the cells. Lifestyle causes us to age quicker, and this is shown in the cells. This is proven by a study of 186 identical twins (4). We decide for ourselves whether we want to slow down our aging process or to repair damage. Our body needs water and protein for this (5). Our body cells consist of up to 85% water. If the cells lose just 10% of water, they age rapidly. This means that the mitochondria (the energy power plants of the cells) are broken down, and the ribosomes (the protein producers of the cells) are also reduced when there is a lack of water. The result: The overall metabolism and cell respiration decrease, the cells shrink and can no longer defend themselves against pathogens, pollutants, and, above all, toxins, and they die off completely over time. We have less energy, are more at risk of obesity and illness and no longer regenerate. This aging process becomes visible very quickly, especially in the skin. The top layer of skin, the epidermis, can absorb three times as much water as it weighs. This allows it to maintain its natural skin protection barrier. Dry skin indicates a lack of water in the body, becomes wrinkled easily, and is prone to inflammation.

WATER - FOOD NO.1 - OUR PERSONAL DRINKING TIPS:

Drinking in everyday life, practical use of living water to maintain good health
– Drink unpolluted, non-carbonated, artesian water
– Drink from glass bottles, avoid PET bottles
– Avoid sweetened liquids
– Take care of your drinking water: it should always be available
– Create water islands at work and privately
– Keep a water-drinking log
– Pass on your knowledge of the truth of water

Our contribution from WATER OF LIFE to AGENDA 2030:
1. We achieve universal and equitable access to quality drinking water.
2. We rely on innovative drinking water logistics with up to 80% CO_2 reduction.
3. We increase the efficiency of water use – avoiding bottle washing.
4. We protect all water-connected ecosystems: mountains, forests, wetlands, rivers, lakes, seas, and aquifers.
5. We support global international WASH projects (Water Sanitary Hygiene).

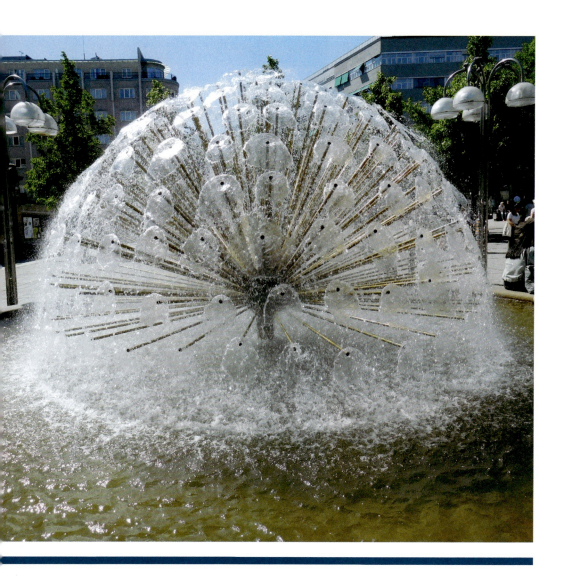

LOOKING INTO A SUSTAINABLE WATER FUTURE

WATER-SMART INDUSTRIES: PRACTICAL APPLICATION, CHALLENGES, AND SOLUTIONS

Geoff Townsend (Industry fellow at NALCO Water)

INTRODUCTION

Industry uses half of all sectoral freshwater in Europe (FAO AQUASTAT). This is more than twice the global average (22%). The distinctive challenges associated with industrial water use are therefore magnified accordingly, making the finding and adoption of solutions to these essential. Three areas in particular warrant special attention – the interrelationship between water and energy (the so-called water-energy nexus), environmental flows, and eutrophication. We will briefly consider each interaction in turn as well as discuss the topic of wetlands where all three converge and potentially have their greatest influence.

Water and energy are business imperatives – strategic resources that enable growth, profitability, and competitiveness of industry. Despite this reality, the rate of growth of water-related risks is far outpacing the efforts being made to mitigate those risks. In 2015, for example, the World Resources Institute projected a 40% gap between fresh water supply and demand by 2030; it has since revised that number to 56% (Luck, Landis, and Gassert, 2015). This ever-widening disparity is attracting the attention of investors, shareholders, and regulators.

It is not simply that more people require more water but rather how the rapidly expanding global middle class is demanding much more water. "During the 20th century, while the population grew by a factor of four, freshwater withdrawals grew by a factor of nine" (Waughray, 2010). If we extrapolate this to 2030, the outlook is stark. Not surprisingly, industrial water use is a major component of this disparity, reflecting the increase in demand for goods that tend to be more water and energy intensive both in their manufacturing and in their use. For example, it takes on average 13,000 litres of water to produce a smart phone. Of note are the rare Earth metals used to manufacture their batteries, magnets, speakers, glass screens, and LED lights (Burley, 2015). Here one tonne of ore generates more than 75,000 litres of acidic wastewater, which is also invariably contaminated with arsenic, barium, cadmium, lead, fluoride, and sulphate.

Then there are the data centres that lie at the heart of our connected world. This industry has "grown from zero in the 1980s, to enabling 60% of the global population to be connected in 2021 via 7.2 million data centres" (Andrews *et al.*, 2021). In most cases the data servers themselves are kept cool by pumping water through the systems, using an equivalent of 120,000 Olympic-sized swimming pools per year. The data centre industry is expected to "grow by around 500% by 2030, as more people and objects are connected via the Internet of Things (IoT)" (Andrews *et al.*, 2021). Key to driving the right behaviour here is the adoption of sustainability indicators including the Water Usage Effectiveness (WUE) indicator to compliment the Power Usage Effectiveness that is already being used to help data centres operate more energy efficiently.

THE WATER-ENERGY NEXUS

We cannot forecast resource requirements accurately without understanding the interconnectivity between resource types. In the past, water, food, and energy were typically dealt with as separate issues. Biofuels epitomise this. Once hailed as a breakthrough for sustainable energy, "bio-diesel's insatiable appetite for wheat" caused spikes in food prices and even led to civil unrest (Smedley, 2013). Global water demand would have also increased by 6 – 7% for only a 10% conversion of fossil fuel to biofuel used for transport (Hoekstra, 2015). This serves to illustrate how vital it is that solutions equally consider the other components of the nexus for water, energy, and food.

Adopting a nexus approach especially highlights the importance of the water-energy component. Water is needed for energy production, and energy is crucial for the provision and treatment of water. The considerable amounts of energy associated with abstracting, pumping, treating, heating, cooling, and cleaning water greatly magnify the impact of industrial water use. When we consider the energy demand of water, pumping is a good place to start as it consumes around a quarter of all electricity on many industrial sites. The overwhelming majority of pumps operate inefficiently. There can be multiple reasons for this, such as being over-sized or having partially worn impellers or motors. Comparing the actual performance with the design pump curve often demonstrates that low-efficiency and/or worn pumps can consume up to 40% more energy than design pumps (World Pumps, 2015).

On the flip side, energy production requires significant inputs of freshwater. In Western Europe, over a third of all abstracted water is used for this purpose. In a conventional thermal power plant, 85 – 95% of the total water needed is for cooling, equating to around 50 billion m^3 of water abstracted in Europe per annum (EEA, 2017). Cooling towers are invariably the largest heat exchangers and the largest consumers of water on industrial sites. Remarkably, more of the intrinsic energy associated with the fuel consumed by thermal power plants is rejected to the cooling system (and consequently the surrounding atmosphere) than is actually converted into electricity. This highlights the importance of cooling system cleanliness, particularly of the condenser, if maximum efficiency is to be attained. The two most common impacts on condenser cleanliness are scale and biofilm formation. Scale formation arises from the deposition of sparingly soluble salts that originate in the water. It characteristically forms a hard crystalline material on the condenser surface. The solubility of the most common scales have an inverse relationship with temperature such that they are more likely to deposit on the hottest part of the heat exchange surface, i.e. the very places where efficient cooling is most critical.

Biofilms are a collective of one or more types of microorganisms that can grow on wet surfaces. Most cooling systems present ideal conditions for microbiological growth, and therefore very close attention has to be paid to this component of the management strategy. Biofilm can have a very pronounced effect on the efficiency of heat transfer, having a thermal conductivity much lower than common scales such as calcium carbonate. Chlorine dioxide is very effective at minimising biofilm growth. An application of this biocide on a cooling system of a 500 MW coal-fired power station reduced the annual carbon dioxide emissions by 50,300 tonnes (equivalent to 22,700 fewer cars on the road) and generated financial savings in excess of €3.1 million per annum, providing a payback period of less than three months. Multiplied across European power production, maximising condenser cleanliness represents an enormous energy saving opportunity (Ecolab, 2018).

We see increasingly that operations cannot adequately decarbonise without understanding the essential role of water. Notably, the most energy intensive industrial operations in Europe (power production, ethylene, oil and gas, steel, etc.) are also very water-intensive, especially in the use of water as an energy transfer medium. Water is ideally suited to this purpose given its high heat capacity – one of the highest of any liquid. In oil refining, for example, between 35 and 47% of the site's total energy is transferred in steam production and cooling water. For conventional power generation we are looking at close to 80%. Here we need data-centric technologies such to uncover actionable insights and create value. It is worth pushing through this additional complexity as the prize of emission reduction is so much greater than can be derived from a simple energy audit.

Digital twins are also a powerful way of providing actionable energy-saving insights across utilities. Ecolab recently developed a digital twin of an ethylene plant in Germany and demonstrated that adopting a water-centric view of energy management realised a 9.9% decrease in energy intensity and a reduction of ~ 40,000 tonnes per annum in emissions.

Adopting the nexus approach highlights how data analytics of industrial processes, water reduction and reuse techniques, and advanced irrigation technologies can strengthen the energy potential while reducing GHG emissions. Not surprisingly, particular attention should be given to the production of steam and hot water, given its high energy intensity. Consequently, reducing blowdown, returning more condensate, boiler tube cleanliness, eliminating steam leaks, and steam trap maintenance are all associated with significant energy savings. It is important to apply technologies that drive efficiency in such operations, recognising that these are inextricably linked to good water management practices.

"The interdependency of water and energy is set to intensify in the coming years, with significant implications for both energy and water security" (IEA, 2016). Currently, water scarcity is somewhat compensated through high-energy reserves and economic power. By 2040, desalination projects will account for 20% of water-related electricity demand (IEA, 2016). Large-scale water transfer projects and an increasing demand for wastewater treatment (or improved treatment processes) also contribute to the water sector's rising energy needs and raises concerns about the potential for fugitive emissions of methane – a powerful greenhouses gas 25 times more potent than carbon dioxide over 100 years (EPA, 2022). These all have significant implications for emissions and growth.

Consequently, it is vital that we better understand the interrelationships between water and climate, not least as water is the primary medium through which we will feel the effects of climate change. Therefore, at the heart of the water-energy nexus is the rapidly growing appreciation that "climate and water systems are linked, and changes in one system induce important, non-linear changes in the other" (World Economic Forum, 2010). Water supply and demand and "energy production have an impact on climate; climate changes affect the availability of water; and the availability of water, in turn, has an effect on energy production" (World Economic Forum, 2010).

Unlike energy supply with its global political and economic dimensions, the availability of water is very much a local issue which will have to be addressed by improved governance at the catchment level. Similarly, the pathway to a low carbon economy could easily exacerbate water stress or be limited by it if it is not properly managed. While "technologies such as wind and solar PV require very little water, others like biofuels production, concentrating solar power, carbon capture and storage (CCS), and nuclear power typically have more significant water demands" (IEA, 2016). In the European Commission Long Term Energy Strategy, hydrogen could account for up to 16-20 % of the total EU energy share (EEB, 2021). However, supplying this equivalent in hydrogen would use about a third of the total water consumed in the energy sector today. This highlights some of the complexity surrounding the impact of decarbonisation strategies.

While most organisations have set clear climate and water goals as part of their 2030 ambition, it is increasingly evident that a large percentage do not have a sufficient plan in place to achieve them. Given the water-energy nexus, an organisations' water and climate strategies need alignment to achieve their full potential.

Most environmental non-governmental organisations (NGO's) maintain that the collapse of biodiversity has potentially even greater impacts than climate change. It is a two-way process. "Climate change is one of the main drivers of biodiversity loss, but the destruction of ecosystems undermines nature's ability to regulate greenhouse gas emissions and protect against extreme weather, thus accelerating climate change and increasing vulnerability to it. This explains why the two crises must be tackled together with holistic policies that address both issues simultaneously and not in silos" (European Commission, 2021). Water is central to this holistic strategy. This brings us on to environmental flows.

ENVIRONMENTAL FLOWS

Environmental flows describe the amount and quality of water that is required to support and sustain freshwater ecosystems and the life that depends on them (including humans). They are vital for healthy aquatic ecosystems, ensure there is a secure supply of drinking water and provide a reliable supply of water for a sustainable economy.

It may not be immediately obvious why environmental flows and industrial water use are connected. Here we need to consider that access to drinking water is a human right and irrigation rights for agriculture are often embedded in local laws that go back centuries. Therefore, in a significant proportion of catchments it is industrial water use that is the 'tail-end' of consumption, dictating how much water is 'left for the environment.' Consequently, there is often a much tighter correlation between industrial water consumption and the environmental flow requirement necessary to sustain aquatic ecosystems compared to the other two sectors (municipal and agriculture). This is particularly the case for sustainable wetlands.

EUTROPHICATION

"Eutrophication is the process by which an entire body of water, or parts of it, becomes progressively enriched with minerals and nutrients" (Wikipedia, 2022). In freshwater ecosystems it is invariably caused by excess phosphorus (Schindler & Vallentyne, 2008), while in coastal waters, the main contributing nutrient is more likely to be nitrogen, or a combination of nitrogen and phosphorus (Elser *et al.*, 2007). This depends on the location and other factors.

Run-off from agricultural land is the main source of nitrogen pollution, whereas households and industry are mostly responsible for phosphorus pollution (although the agricultural contribution can be up to 40% in areas of intensive farming). Over the past 20 years, phosphorus concentrations have fallen in many river systems, mainly driven by upgrading wastewater treatment plants to include phosphorus removal. The significant shift to phosphate-free detergents has also contributed. Industry needs to continue these reductions in phosphate discharge as it is still widely used as a corrosion inhibitor in cooling systems. The latter also commonly uses phosphorus-containing phosphonates as scale inhibitors. Here moving to non-phosphate alternatives minimise the risk of eutrophication and the impact that it can have on freshwater biodiversity. It is also vital to have high awareness of emerging threats to biodiversity such as PFASs, engineered nanomaterials, and microplastic pollution.

WETLANDS

Wetlands are where water, climate, and biodiversity most strongly converge. Wetlands are highly efficient at capturing carbon. "Freshwater peatlands cover only 3% of global land surface but store twice as much carbon (550Gt) as all the planet's forests combined (WWT, 2019). Tragically they are also being lost at three times the rate of forests, leading to the release of methane and nitrous oxides greenhouse gases with a far stronger global warming potential than carbon dioxide" (GIZ, 2020, Reuters, 2020). There is a case that carbon offsetting via water may be more important than the current practise of planting trees. "More than 10% of annual carbon dioxide emissions result from the degradation and destruction of peat swamps" (Butler, 2007). 90% of Europe's wetlands are gone, so the focus should be on large-scale restoration. 84% of freshwater species are in decline worldwide (WWF, 2020). Overall, "40% of the world's species are reliant in some way on wetlands, so the loss of these valuable places is forcing many species to the brink of extinction" (WWT, 2021).
"Environmental allocations are not only intended to maintain biodiversity and aquatic ecology but are recognised as vital to ensuring the continuing provision of environmental goods and services upon which peoples' lives and livelihoods depend" (WWF, 2007).

In addition to being a vital natural carbon sink, wetlands act as a natural buffer against the most extreme events, soaking up heavy rainfall and ameliorating water flows. "As well as being threatened by pollution, wetlands also have an important role in addressing it. They can act as natural filters, helping to remove pollutants from the water (they have the potential to remove up to 60% of metals, trap and retain up to 90% of sediment runoff and eliminate up to 90% of nitrogen)" (WWT, 2020a, 2020b). One cannot say that sustainable water use has been achieved at a particular location unless wetlands have the environmental flows they need to support biodiversity and carbon sequestration. It is likely that in many catchments across Europe, the benefit of reducing water consumption on environmental carbon capture is greater than the emissions we save via the direct applications of energy-saving technologies. It is very important to be aware of this as consumptive water targets are set for the industry.

DEVELOPING AN INDUSTRIAL WATER STRATEGY

Creating a robust water security plan for an industrial site requires a comprehensive risk and opportunity mapping exercise. Both aspects are vital considerations with potentially a lot at stake if key elements are overlooked. In 2020, across all sectors, the Carbon Disclosure Project (CDP) stated that companies reported the maximum financial impacts of water risks at US$301 billion – five times higher than the cost of addressing them (US$55 billion) (CDP, 2021a). Not only does risk mitigation provide an impressive return, it is also important to recognise the considerable extent to which water creates societal value – it enables growth and competitive advantage. CDP also stated that beyond risk management, there are business opportunities when investing in water security – estimated at US$711 billion.

Water risks are frequently categorised as physical, regulatory, and reputational. The financial impacts associated with these are wide-ranging from revenue loss and supply chain disruption to higher energy and capital costs.

"Water pricing typically bears no relation to how scarce water is or the realities on the ground," Alexis Morgan, WWF (Klein, 2022). "Unlike most commodities, there are very few free markets to set water prices according to supply and demand dynamics" (Lynagh, 2022). In fact, globally there is an inverse relationship between water stress (and its associated risk) and its unit price. Consequently, if only the latter is used in return-on-investment calculations for risk mitigation, then it is highly likely that the organisation will continue to be exposed to considerable financial impacts.

Ecolab's Smart Water Navigator (Ecolab, 2022) is a free public platform that uses an algorithm that considers "biodiversity, environmental issues, ecosystem services, health impacts, and recreational services to calculate a premium for the local water price that accurately reflects the actual cost of using the water" (Klein, 2022). "The tool has been very popular with ESG investors, who use it when evaluating a company's proposed new facility location or development. For example, for a site in Bangalore, the current water bill price is just 21 cents per cubic meter. But according to the Smart Water Navigator's risk calculations, the price should be $2.62" (Klein, 2022).

The Smart Water Navigator can also be used to set meaningful, localised targets (Figure 1). In addition, "*Setting Site Water Targets Informed by Catchment Context:*

A Guide for Companies," published by the CEO Water Mandate (CEO Water Mandate, 2019) provides a useful framework here. It is also helpful to align targets with global environmental standards set by respected organisations, such as the Global Reporting Initiative (GRI), Sustainability Accounting Standards Board (SASB), and the Carbon Disclosure Project (CDP).

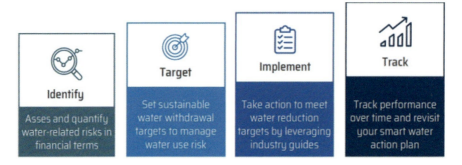

Figure 1. The Ecolab Smart Water Navigator uses a proven, four-step process to enhance business resilience at all levels of an organisation through smart water management.

Based on geographic location, water risk assessment tools generate basin and sub-basin data on water risks. Facility risks are then aggregated to rank a company's overall water risk exposure. This analysis may be supplemented by operational data, such as production or water withdrawals, and may be extended to a company's value chain. A deeper dive into local/operational water risks is then recommended by industry bodies such as the CEO Water Mandate (CEO Water Mandate, 2019), followed by an analysis around the six shared water challenges aligned with the Sustainable Development Goal (SDG) 6, 11.5, and 13.1 targets: 1) access to safe water, sanitation, and hygiene (WASH); 2) water quality; 3) water quantity; 4) water governance; 5) important water-related ecosystems; and 6) extreme weather events (CEO Water Mandate, 2019).

Water risk assessments are not only valuable for businesses to understand their risk and impacts, but they are also valuable for other local stakeholders in the same regions. This can include NGOs, governments, municipal utilities, indigenous peoples, and local communities who also rely on the ongoing health of shared water basins.

"Barclays analysts estimate that 19 – 27 % of industrial withdrawals are from areas with high or extremely high water risk" (Klein, 2022). Here industry often pays a hugely subsidised cost for water. Not surprisingly, investors are urging greater transparency and action from companies regarding these risks. In 2021, over 590 investors with over US$110 trillion in assets requested companies to disclose on water security impacts, risks, and actions through CDP's platform (CDP, 2021a, 2021b).

Consequently, even in the face of climate change, resilient businesses are those that identify, monetise, and mitigate water-related risks in a cost-proportionate way, while appreciating that water is a fundamental enabler of value creation. Key to building such resiliency is ensuring that the impacts on water resources are within the capacity of the local catchment. This is vital as to date water reduction activity has been largely self-determined rather than setting robust and meaningful water targets that take into account the unique local contexts of the basins in which companies operate. These Context Based Water Targets (CBWT's), as they are known, are considered the most credible indicator of sustainable water use and therefore the level of exposure to risk at a given locality.

Setting Context-Based Water Targets is not a quick process, as the WWF recently pointed out (Dobson & Morgan, 2018), but they are potentially the last targets needed to be set as they highlight the finish line, not the next benchmark.

Once the destination is known, one can set about planning the journey, producing the frameworks and deploying the technologies that ensure that a production site's performance is within the capacity of the basin's renewable supply of water and ability to assimilate pollutants.

"In a world that is set to face ongoing water quantity and quality challenges, CBWTs are all about working towards an end state that ensures long-term business viability for operations and supply chains" (Dobson & Morgan, 2018).

The current inability to adequately determine the sustainable use of water at a particular location represents one of the greatest obstacles to progress in water management and its stewardship. Most of the time companies have no idea what they are aiming for. There is no clear sustainability "end point": In its absence we keep hearing "our goal is to be 20% more efficient," what forever? That's not going to work!

This absence of a clear process for quantifying sustainable water use is exacerbating the several challenges industries face such as "a lack of established governance systems, weak participatory processes, and the difficulty of getting internal high-level commitments" and investments to secure their water future (WBCSD, 2013).

These factors serve to highlight the complexity of water derived from it being a local, finite, and shared resource. On top of this, it can have high temporal variability, its quality can change very quickly, and it has "social, environmental, and economic uses that are each valued differently by its users" (Dobson & Morgan, 2018).

In addition to the challenges in determining whether water use is sustainable or not, this complexity can also make it difficult to assess at any given time how to maximise performance from water. This is very relevant to industrial water use where we put "water to work" as a process fluid for heating and cooling, etc.

The enormity and complexity of these challenges is only being tempered by the pace of technological development. This is why developing and deploying a digitalisation strategy for water is so critical. Harnessing the rapid advancements in technology is our only hope to adequately deal with the complexity of water as a shared resource.

As the water crisis looms large, there is a danger of focussing too much on advocating solutions to the neglect of being able to characterise the level of water performance that is needed to be achieved now and in the future. Innovation that supports the robust quantification of sustainable water use will, in turn, drive the breakthrough innovations in water saving or enabling technologies that we still need. The one flows from the other.

Until we fully grasp the magnitude of the gap between actual and sustainable water use, we cannot determine whether we are under or over-investing in enabling technologies nor will we be able to truly calculate the value they create and their return on investment. Underpinning all this is the key requisite of confidence. Confidence in the framework, the algorithms, the economic evaluations of 'value add' and, of course, the data.

Without a high level of confidence, there will not be the significant investments necessary to reduce, reuse, and/or recycle the volumes of water required to achieve sustainable water use. This connectivity between confidence and achieving sustainable water use is clear.

What are these innovations that are so crucial to our understanding of sustainable water use and our ability to achieve it?

The first is the need for catchment-level insights to manage water risk. It is recommended that a so-called 'layered approach' is adopted as this should enable inclusiveness and upgradability at each layer. The foundational 'layer' is a catchment map, upon which abstraction points can be positioned, potentially highlighting the 'sub-catchment' per abstraction point. Upon this up-to-date rainfall data can be superimposed from the considerable number of weather stations already connected to the internet. Where applicable, a similar approach can be used to capture ground water levels.
Satellite imagery and other forms of earth observation, combined with remote sensing, IoT, Artificial Intelligence (AI), and other advanced technologies can increasingly enable accurate quantification of evapotranspiration rates associated with land use as well as soil moisture levels (WEF, 2018). Such technologies enable us to detect water basin risks much earlier. For example, satellite models already exist that correlate soil moisture with recent rainfall in order to detect areas of overirrigation.

Secondly, a variety of tools are being developed that enable the quantification and communication of water risk (Ecolab, 2022), and then identify and implement solutions to manage it accordingly. These include technologies that disseminate common catchment goals and thereby help communicate the local water management ambition. In turn, this can help drive the cooperation and collaboration between local stakeholders – a vital component of a robust water stewardship strategy, especially in water stressed areas.

Thirdly, "blockchain-based technology could fundamentally transform the way water resources are managed and traded" (WEF, 2018) by providing a secure, transparent, and distributed ledger to record transactions between parties (Stinson, 2018, WEF 2018).

Such radical transparency is much needed, reducing the risk of corruption and potentially reducing the information asymmetry that can blight water management. Crucially, this could enable everyone and anyone from individuals, farmers, industry consumers, water managers, and policymakers to access the same data on water quality and quantity and make more informed decisions (Stinson, 2018).

"Blockchain technology could also support peer-to-peer trading of water rights/ allocations in a given catchment, empowering water users who have enough or are willing to share their excess resources with others in the area to do so 24/7 without relying on a centralised authority" (Stinson, 2018, WEF 2018). This is very much aligned to the stakeholder inclusive process that sits at the heart of water stewardship principles.

"This type of transparent, real-time approach to water management could greatly mitigate tensions within and across certain localities by democratising access to information and preventing the tampering of data" (WEF 2018).

Fourthly, innovation that supports the so-called "3'R's" – technologies that reduce, reuse, or recycle water can be decentralised or form part of an integrated water reuse system. Either way, their deployment should be commensurate with the internal efficiency or quality objectives needed to achieve the local catchment context-based targets. Crucially these technologies need to be reliable, consistently delivering the required performance despite the inherent challenges of treating water.

As we move toward a circular economy, wastewater needs to be considered as a valuable resource rather than a liability. Success here is predicated on understanding the true value IN water whether that be embedded energy, metals, or nutrients.

Only 3% of wastewater is reclaimed today – the impact of increasing this to 10% would be enormous. New technologies are enabling wastewater to be used directly in cooling systems. However, without proper management, wastewater can increase the risk of reliability impacts on such systems whether these be from localised corrosion or excessive microbiological growth. This highlights the importance of understanding the interrelationships between efficiency and reliability, as shown graphically below (Figure 2).

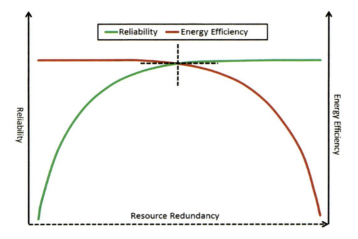

Figure 2. Reliability and Energy Efficiency Trade-off (After Sharma et al., 2016).

Here, 'optimum' is typically a moving target given the often-considerable variability in the driving forces for both factors.

Ecolab's 3D TRASAR™ technology captures the necessary insights to achieve this optimum consistently (Ecolab, 2021). It continuously monitors and controls water-intensive processes and collects and analyses the data in real time, providing actionable intelligence that can be used to benchmark performance and drive continuous improvement. Nearly 40,000 of these systems have been deployed on cooling systems globally, collecting and analysing real-time water usage data to improve efficiency and cut water, energy, and operational costs. 3D TRASAR technology has saved so much water, a counter to keep track of these savings has been included on the technology's webpage. In 2021, it helped conserve 605,422,725 m^3 of water, equivalent to the annual drinking water needs of more than 552.2 million people.

Each unit is tied to a location providing an important local context to these systems given they are typically the largest users of water on industrial sites. Shared through the cloud, the data is accessible to Ecolab service personnel through mobile devices.

Finally, there is a need for innovative finance solutions and business models that leverage digital technologies enabling them to be deployed at scale and the collective resilience that would provide.

In conclusion, if we cannot quantify location-specific sustainable water use and determine its value socially, environmentally, and economically how can we develop an adequate understanding of the impacts of population growth, climate change, urbanisation, land use change or the much needed insights into the water-energy-food nexus?

Action to address these does not yet match the urgency or scale of the challenges. A different approach is needed. Rylan Dobson and Alexis Morgan (WWF) capture this succinctly: "The global/local trends of supply and demand imbalances that most basins face will not be resolved by setting more "ambitious" efficiency targets. We collectively face a choice: (1) businesses continue to set incremental internal efficiency related targets, and put everyone's assets at risk, or (2) businesses embrace this new normal, and engage in fundamentally shifting corporate water target paradigms that will maintain key thresholds of sustainability and enable all to thrive" (Dobson & Morgan, 2018).

REFERENCES

Andrews, D., Newton, E., Adibi, N., Chenadec, J. and Bienge, K. (2021). A Circular Economy for the Data Centre Industry: Using Design Methods to Address the Challenge of Whole System Sustainability in a Unique Industrial Sector. Sustainability 2021, 13, 6319.

Burley, H. (2015). Mind your step – The land and water footprints of everyday products. Friends of the Earth.

Butler, R.A. (2007), https://news.mongabay.com/2007/12/10-of-global-co2-emissions-result-from-swamp-destruction/ 10 December 2007.

CDP, (2021a). Carbon Disclosure Project. Cost of water risks to business five times higher than cost of taking action. Carbon Disclosure Project, 19 March 2021.

CDP (2021b). Carbon Disclosure Project. 2% of companies worldwide worth $12 trillion named on CDP's A List of environmental leaders. Carbon Disclosure Project, 7 December 2021.

CEO Water Mandate (2019). Setting Site Water Targets Informed by Catchment Context: A Guide for Companies. UN Global Compact CEO Water Mandate, Pacific Institute, CDP, The Nature Conservancy, World Resources Institute, WWF, UNEPDHI Partnership Centre for Water and Environment. 2019.

Dobson, R and Morgan, A (2018). Context-Based Water Targets: Why should business care? 20 August 2018. https://wwf.medium.com/context-based-water-targets-why-should-business-care-561bd82a90f7

EEA (2017). European Environment Agency. Use of freshwater resources in Europe. https://www.eea.europa.eu/data-and-maps/indicators/use-of-freshwater-resources-3/assessment-4.

EEB (2021). Face to face with hydrogen – The reality behind the hype. European Environmental Bureau, May 2021.

Ecolab Inc. (2018). CH2061E – Nalco Water's OMNI offering helps a Northern European customer save 3 Million Euros per year.

Ecolab Inc. (2021). https://en-uk.ecolab.com/offerings/3d-trasar-technology-for-cooling-water

Ecolab Inc. (2022). https://en-uk.ecolab.com/corporate-responsibility/environment/water-stewardship/smart-water-navigator

Elser, J., Bracken, M., Cleland, E., Gruner, D., Harpole, W., Hillebrand, H., Ngai, J., Seabloom, E., Shurin, J. and Smith, J. (2007). "Global analysis of nitrogen and phosphorus limitation of primary producers in freshwater, marine and terrestrial ecosystems". Ecology Letters. 10 (12): 1135–1142.

EPA (2022). U.S. Environmental Protection Agency. https://www.epa.gov/gmi/importance-methane 9th June 2022.

European Commission (2021). https://ec.europa.eu/research-and-innovation/en/horizon-magazine/climate-change-and-biodiversity-loss-should-be-tackled-together.

FAO (2018). Food and Agriculture Organisation of the United Nations, AQUASTAT database, 2018.

GIZ (2020). Stop Floating, Start Swimming. Deutsche Gesellschaft für Internationale Zusammenarbeit (GIZ) GmbH.

Google. Environmental Report 2019. Tech. Rep., Google. https://services.google.com/fh/files/misc/google_2019-environmental-report.pdf (2020).

Hoekstra, A. (2015). Switching to biofuels could place unsustainable demands on water use. Guardian Sustainable Business, 28 May 2015.

IEA (2016). International Energy Agency. A delicate balance between water demand and the low-carbon energy transition, 15 November 2016. https://www.iea.org/news/a-delicate-balance-between-water-demand-and-the-low-carbon-energy-transition.

Klein, J. (2022). Will water pricing be the next carbon pricing? GreenBiz 101. https://www.greenbiz.com/article/will-water-pricing-be-next-carbon-pricing

Luck, M., Landis, M. and Gassert, F. (2015). "Aqueduct Water Stress Projections: Decadal Projections of Water Supply and Demand Using CMIP5 GCMs." Technical Note. Washington, D.C.: World Resources Institute.

Lynagh, C, (2020) Industrial Equipment & Technology industries. https://www.morganstanley.com/ideas/water-scarcity-causes-and-solutions

OECD. OECD Environmental Outlook to 205 (OECD Publishing, 2012). https://doi.org/10.1787/9789264122246-en.

Le Moal M., Gascuel-Odoux C., Ménesguen A., Souchon Y., Étrillard C., Levain A., Moatar F., Pannard A., Souchu P., Lefebvre A. and Pinay G. (2019). "Eutrophication: A new wine in an old bottle?" Science of the Total Environment. 651 (Pt 1): 1–11.

Reuters Events (2020). https://www.reutersevents.com/sustainability/connecting-drops-battle-against-climate-change

Schindler, D. and Vallentyne, J. (2008). The Algal Bowl: Overfertilization of the World's Freshwaters and Estuaries, University of Alberta Press, ISBN 0-88864-484-1.

Sharma, Y., Javadi, B., Si, W., and Sun, D.W. (2016). Reliability and energy efficiency in cloud computing systems: Survey and taxonomy. J. Netw. Comput. Appl., 74, 66-85.

Smedley, T. (2013). Securing a sustainable future. The Guardian Sustainable Food. Nexus Live Debates. 22 Feb 2013.

Stinson, C. (2018). How blockchain, AI and other emerging technologies could end water insecurity. GreenBiz, April 2, 2018. https://www.greenbiz.com/article/how-blockchain-ai-and-other-emerging-technologies-could-end-water-insecurity

Waughray, D. (2010). Why worry about water? A quick global overview. Guardian Sustainable Business, 10 November 2010.

WBCSD (2013). The World Business Council for Sustainable Development. Sharing Water: Engaging Business, 11 April 2013.

Wikipedia (2022). https://en.wikipedia.org/wiki?curid=54840

WEF (2018). World Economic Forum. 5 ways the Fourth Industrial Revolution could end water insecurity, 22 March 2018.

World Economic Forum (2010). Thirsty Energy: Water and Energy in the 21st Century. Published 24 October 2010.

World Pumps (2015). Energy efficient pumps help fight climate change. 20th Aug 2015. https://www.worldpumps.com/content/features/energy-efficient-pumps-help-fight-climate-change

WWF (2007). World Wildlife Fund. Allocating Scarce Water. April 2007.

WWF (2020). World Wildlife Fund. 84% collapse in Freshwater species populations since 1970. 10 September 2020. https://wwf.panda.org/wwf_news/?804991/84-collapse-in-Freshwater-species-populations-since-1970

WWT (2019). Wildfowl & Wetlands Trust. Climate change and wetlands – How wetlands could help solve the climate change problem. https://www.wwt.org.uk/our-work/threats-to-wetlands/climate-change-and-wetlands/, May 2019.

WWT (2020a). Wildfowl & Wetlands Trust. Why wetlands? Incredible things happen when land and water meet, June 2020. https://www.wwt.org.uk/our-work/why-wetlands/

WWT (2020b). Wildfowl & Wetlands Trust. https://www.wwt.org.uk/our-work/threats-to-wetlands

WWT (2021). Wildfowl & Wetlands Trust. Wetlands for nature and people – Creating a world where healthy wetland nature thrives and enriches lives, June 2021.

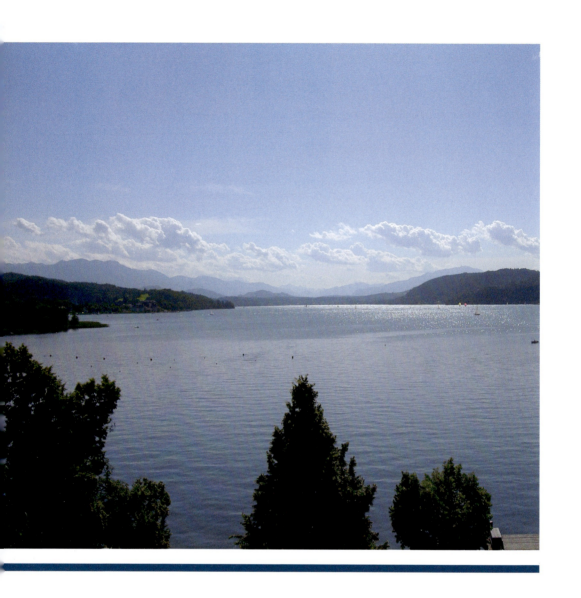

WATER & PUBLIC HEALTH

Cristian Carboni (Industrie De Nora S.p.a.), Marianna Brichese

Water is vital for human health. In 2010, the UN General Assembly explicitly recognised the human right to water and sanitation[1] and on July 28th, 2022, the UN General Assembly declared access to a clean, healthy, and sustainable environment a universal human right[2]. The minimum required amount of water for life is around 2.3 litres per day. It means that one should be guaranteed the access to this quantity of water. But to ensure the health and wellbeing of communities, the access to water should be broader. Together with the quantity, also the quality of water needs to be ensured.

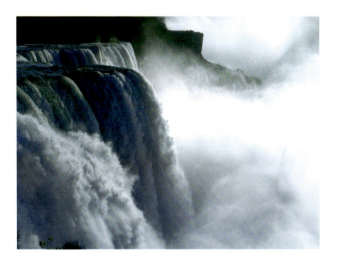

Water and the good hygiene habits associated with it allow to reduce the spread of some diseases: for example, we have seen the importance of washing and sanitising hands around the world to counter the spread of SARS-CoV-2 or to reduce diarrhea in developing countries. Water, however, impacts human life also indirectly due to its uses to produce food, energy, and to process goods and materials. In addition, water is closely linked to the ecosystems in which we live and with which we are interconnected, being therefore critical to our health and the ecosystem, too.

Today, however, the availability of clean and safe water is still precluded for many people. To ensure public health, the main challenges to be addressed are water scarcity, microbiological threats, and the presence of residues. These issues are exacerbated by climate change: the long-term effects of climate change, with higher intensity rainfall, may influence the degree of environmental impacts caused by the intermittent discharges and runoff events. Pollution events may become more frequent, spilling greater volumes. The overall challenge is to ensure access to safe water for all but in an environmentally sustainable way.

1   World Health Organization 2019: Safer water, better health. 2019 update
2   WHO, UNICEF: Progress on Drinking Water, Sanitation and Hygiene

Water scarcity issues have been addressed in previous chapters; we will focus on the main aspects related to water quality.

MICROBIOLOGICAL RISK

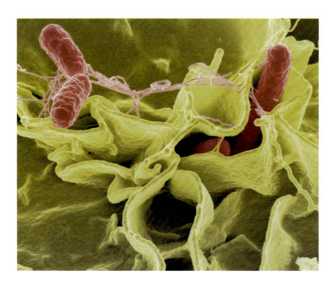

Infectious disease caused by poor microbiological water can generate outbreaks. This is the starting point for severe epidemics, if there is the case of lack of control of its diffusion. A large proportion of the overall disease burden, 3.3% of global deaths and 4.6% of global disability-adjusted life years (DALYs), was attributed to the quantifiable effects of inadequate water, sanitation, and hygiene (WASH) in 2016[3]. This represents nearly 2 million preventable deaths and 123 million preventable DALYs annually. Even in developed countries, there are infections caused by pathogens transmitted through water, and problems of resistance to disinfectants and antibiotics emerge. Water-borne diseases include viral hepatitis, typhoid, cholera, dysentery, and other diseases that cause diarrhea. Campylobacteriosis, giardiasis, hepatitis A, and shigellosis are the most commonly reported gastrointestinal infectious diseases in the WHO European Region; diseases with the highest number of reported outbreaks are viral gastroenteritis, hepatitis A, E. coli, diarrhoea, and legionellosis. (WHO 2016). In particular *Legionella* bacteria can spread in pipelines during out-of-use periods and then be diffused by aerosol in showers, evaporative towers, irrigation, and AC systems, causing severe diseases. Water-based diseases and water-related vector-borne diseases can result from water supply projects, including dams and irrigation structures that inadvertently provide habitats for

---

3   World Health Organization 2016: The situation of water-related infectious diseases in the pan-European region

mosquitoes and snails that are intermediate hosts of the parasites that cause malaria, schistosomiasis, lymphatic filariasis, onchocerciasis, and Japanese encephalitis.

Microorganisms in the water, however, not only cause direct harm but can also produce toxins, such as those produced by some varieties of algae. Excess nutrient inputs can indeed lead to eutrophication in surface waters, a process characterised by increased plant growth, problem algal blooms, loss of life in the bottom water, and an undesirable disturbance to the balance of organisms present in the water.

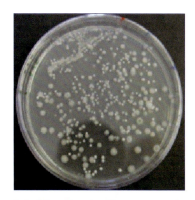

In addition, the microbiological risk is exacerbated by water shortages and extreme weather phenomena related to climate change: supply disruptions, as well as floods and inundations, can provide the ideal breeding grounds for bacteria and pathogens.

The last but very impacting point is also the presence of a high quantity of antibiotics in waste water, increasing the antibiotic-resistance trouble. Antimicrobial resistance is considered be the next global emergency (UN 2019)[4].

WATER CONTAMINANTS AND EMERGING POLLUTANTS

Another main challenge we have to face to guarantee access to safe water for all is emerging pollutants, that is chemicals and compounds that have recently been identified as dangerous to the environment and consequently to the health of human beings.

To achieve the SDG 6 target 6.3 – improve water quality by reducing pollution, halving the proportion of untreated wastewater, and substantially increasing recycling and the safe reuse of water – water pollutants must be measured and reduced to a safe level.

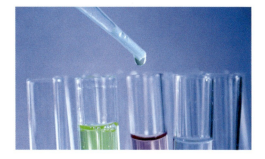

4   Statement of WHO chief Tedros Adhanom Ghebreyesus, 18 June 2019

Examples of contaminants are disinfection byproducts, drugs, endocrine disruptors, toxins, heavy metals, and synthetic chemicals, including fertilisers and pesticides. Drinking water supplies that contain high amounts of certain chemicals, like arsenic and nitrates, can cause serious disease. Arsenic is still a major issue in many countries, like Italy, together with other pollutants such as Fluoride, Nitrates, and Perfluoroalkyl chemicals (PFAS). Nutrients can cause water pollution, too. The most important sources contributing to Biochemical Oxygen Demand (BOD) are domestic wastewaters and industrial wastewater (for example paper or food processing industries) and agriculture with silage effluents and manure. In addition to nutrient and organic pollution, there are many Emerging Pollutants (EPs), also known as Contaminants of Emerging Concern (CECs) that are the substances released into the environment for which no regulations are currently established. They are many organic compounds present as pharmaceuticals and personal care products, hormones, food additives, pesticides, plasticisers, wood preservatives, laundry detergents, disinfectants, surfactants, flame retardants, and other organic compounds in water are mainly generated by human activities.

Furthermore, problems relating to microplastics are urgently emerging. Microplastics are plastic with sizes from 0.1 micron to 5 millimeters, and consist of two types: primary, when released in the environment with those sizes like in the case of residuals from washing machines or the consumption of pneumatics, and secondary, when they are the results of the erosion of bigger plastic items released in the environment. In both cases, one of the most dangerous events is the spread of microplastics in the sea or in other water sources. Techniques to recover and recycle this material are under investigation by research.

POTENTIAL SOLUTIONS

Clearly, it is not possible to formulate a ranking of treatments that is of general validity. Each solution has advantages and disadvantages that must be evaluated in the specific application context, considering multiple factors, providing a preventive risk analysis and a technical-economic-environmental analysis. Conversely, it is well established that only with the integration of multiple processes, and with a complementary spectrum of action, it is possible to achieve a satisfactory level of removal of micropollutants from wastewater.

The choice of processes and the order in which they are arranged depends on multiple factors: the chemical and physical characteristics of the contaminants to be removed; the typical removal principle of each process; the multiplicity of contaminants present and their relative concentration, which can lead to interactions that reduce the efficiency of the processes themselves.

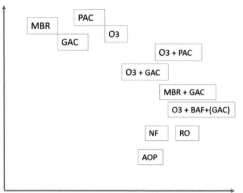

Suitability to Waste Water Treatment Plant

AOP: Advanced Oxidation Process
BAF: Biologically Activated Filter
GAC = Granular Activated Carbon
MBR: Membrane Biofilm Reactor
NF: Nanofiltration
O3 = Ozone
PAC: Powered Activated Carbon
RO: Reverse Osmosis

Range of Pollutants Removed

Alongside primary mechanical treatments, effective secondary biological treatments have been developed. Biological wastewater treatment significantly reduces biodegradable pollution in wastewater and therefore has a direct influence on the surface water quality. Secondary treatment can be an available and effective solution for problems related to high levels of BOD, and for this reason it is necessary to develop and connect as many people as possible to secondary treatment systems even with decentralised systems to be placed in rural areas.

Lastly, tertiary treatments, sometimes called "effluent polishing", are advanced filtration systems that can be used to remove particulate matter. Wastewater may still have high levels of nutrients such as nitrogen and phosphorus, dyes, surfactants, EPs, or other substances that are difficult to degrade by secondary treatment systems. Phosphorus and nitrogen can be removed biologically in a process called enhanced biological phosphorus removal, nitrification, and denitrification. There are also physical/chemical processes to enhance performance by also removing phosphorus and solids in a single-stage process. The removal of arsenic can instead be carried out using a ferric oxide arsenic removal media. The media also adsorbs antimony, cadmium, chromate, lead, molybdenum, selenium, and vanadium. Other systems can remove fluoride onto solid activated alumina.

Concerning the removal of unwanted coloring substances, odours, flavours, and recalcitrant Chemical Oxygen Demand (COD) in the water, excellent results have been obtained employing advanced ozonation or oxidation processes.

Ozone generator

It should be emphasised that the majority of plants, both potabilisation and sewage treatment plants weren't designed specifically for the removal of Emerging Micropollutants (EMs).

The most studied processes in recent decades, applicable at full scale, that are found to be capable of removing EMs are:
− separation on pressurised membranes: Nanofiltration (NF) and Reverse Osmosis (RO);
− adsorption on activated carbon, either in granular (Granular Activated Carbon, GAC) or powdered form or exchange resins (Powdered Activated Carbon, PAC);
− oxidation by ozone or by Advanced Oxidation Processes (AOP).

Membrane separation systems then involve the disposal of concentrates and may require the installation of pretreatment systems to reduce fouling and scaling. Membrane separation systems under pressure not only remove EPs but also salts and therefore should be coupled with remineralisation systems, particularly in drinking water treatment. In addition, the operating costs for large water flows are very high.

Activated carbon processes involve the need for regeneration or disposal of GAC and have poor selectivity toward EPs when competing with other organic compounds. In this sense (reduce disposal), electrooxidation processes are being investigated for the destruction of some pollutants and the regeneration of some resins. AOP can lead to the creation of unmeasurable or unmeasured byproducts, and for this reason, their combination with adsorption systems (such as activated carbon) or membrane systems is often recommended.
An effective combination is ozone and Biological Activated Carbon (BAC), resulting in simultaneous adsorption and biodegradation of organic compounds, or combinations of ozone with Biological Activated Filter (BAF).

This solution is effective when the ozonation stage is well managed, as there are two opposite effects:
− oxidation by ozone usually increases the biodegradability of molecules by enhancing their biodegradation by the biomass attached to the activated carbon granules, which is particularly useful in reducing the organic matter competition for active sites;
− increase in biodegradability usually corresponds to a decrease in the affinity between molecules and activated carbon, reducing the extent of adsorption and prolonging the useful life of the activated carbon.

This type of system is one of the most promising and sustainable.
As can be seen, the solutions often come from a combination of several technologies.

Micropollutants: combination of the most used technologies

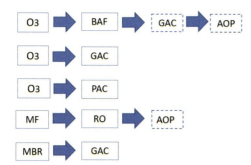

AOP: Advanced Oxidation Process
BAF: Biologically Activated Filter
GAC = Granular Activated Carbon
MBR: Membrane Biofilm Reactor
MF: Microfiltration
O3 = Ozone
PAC: Powered Activated Carbon
RO: Reverse Osmosis

To date, adsorption on activated carbon and ozonation, in addition to biological treatment, has proved to be effective and sustainable from an economic point of view, as demonstrated by the installations in Switzerland and Germany (the latter with the largest number of plants designed to remove micropollutants: about 20 installations). In Austria, pilot-scale trials are underway on ozonation followed by a biological activated carbon filter, in anticipation of a widespread application scale in the near future. Also in other countries, such as France and the Netherlands, the opportunity to equip existing plants with ozonation or activated carbon adsorption treatments is being considered.

Regarding the control of disinfection by-products and, in particular, those indicated by the drinking water directive (such as chlorites and chlorates), there are solutions on the market capable of producing the active ingredients on-site and capable of producing few chlorates. There are also combinations of technologies that make it possible to reduce the disinfection by-products, for example by acting on organic substances and their reaction with oxidising agents. We believe that these solutions are valid because they do not allow for the complete modification of the active ingredients used today for purification (mainly chlorine-based) until complete data are available on the possibility of using other types of active ingredients on a real scale.

If the chlorination process is producing trihalomethanes or haloacetic acids, switching to chlorine dioxide, acting on organic load, making multiple injection points, and other solutions may help solve this problem. Chlorates produced by using bulk hypochlorite can be reduced by switching to on-site low chlorate hypochlorite generation.

Managing wastewater, however, is not only a public health duty and commitment: it is also an opportunity to prevent other problems and know in detail the health status of the population. Recently, techniques of wastewater analysis have been opening new frontiers in the field of epidemiology. Water can be used as an indicator of the population's health level. Wastewater analysis is a promising tool for detecting pathogens, such as the virus SARS-CoV-2 and monitoring the consumption of drugs, medication, etc. Water is therefore strategic for the prevention and understanding of health troubles. The European Union is showing increasing interest in these new frontiers, for example with the COVID-19 Sentinel Programme of the European Commission.

TOWARD A CULTURAL CHANGE

What emerges is that many problem-solving technologies are already available, nevertheless, the research task of developing increasingly sustainable solutions remains important. Available tecnhonologies have not been implemented for lack of regulatory obligations and for budget reasons, as will be made clearer in the next chapters. Therefore, it is necessary to act on the regulatory issue and equip the actors with the appropriate financial resources, either through public funds or through changes in tariff policies. Promoting sustainable financing to deliver and sustain infrastructures and services will be an effective tool. In fact, water safety is not only a matter of pushing technologies: the investments of governments in those technologies must also be pushed, keeping in mind the central role of water issues and the sustainability of all the processes involved. National, European, and international regulations should keep this direction to simplify, harmonise, and facilitate the diffusion of good quality water everywhere.

A radical change in vision is also needed to move from just transposing regulatory parameters to punctual risk analysis. Only in this way will it be possible to identify specific risks and solutions and to contextualise each solution inside a particular ecosystem. In doing so, the concept of exposome will also have to become central in evaluating and making decisions. Science has identified the exposome as an important way to find out the reasons for some diseases and therefore to take of human health. The exposome is the analysis of all of the environmental components people get in contact with during their lifetime. Tracking the place where people lived, air breathed, and water drank, together with the natural or synthetic substances dissolved, helps to lead to the origin of health troubles, and, together with gene map analysis, to complete the puzzle of understanding of some specific diseases. It is important that this personalised approach also takes gender diversity and disability into account, particularly in the design of sanitation and disinfection services.

Ensuring access to clean water and health also requires the involvement of all stakeholders, including end users. Experience shows that constructing water supply and sanitation facilities is not enough to improve health; sanitation and hygiene promotion must accompany the infrastructure investments to realise their full potential as a public health intervention. Water is used by everyone, and if we want to address and structurally solve its problems and spread best practices, including hygienic ones, we must involve everyone, and create widespread responsibility and leadership. Responsive citizens, knowing the preciousness of water, working on consumption and pollution reduction, sensibilisation, and education are the real gold mine for the future.

Thinking in a "Montessori way," education of citizens starts teaching children the sense of responsibility, the importance of repairing damages, and being ready to interact in the real world from a young age. Until now too many people have thought that they are living in a "world for free" where what they do not have an impact on others.

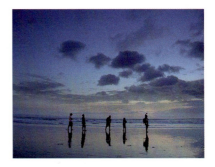

School health programmes offer a good entry point for improved water supply and sanitation facilities and community hygiene promotion, but even more structured and ambitious projects are possible: an example could be the model proposed by the Social Engagement Platform (SEP), a workstream of the UN-World Water Quality Alliance alliance that seeks to promote transparent, multi-stakeholder processes for water management. The objective is to create mutual trust between all social sectors leading to a broad awareness of global and local water issues. The workstream plans to use an approach to provide a simple, realistic, and economically modest roadmap; global problems find supranational, national, regional, and local solutions engaging all members of society. Complex systems are translated to simple language, and data to knowledge and knowledge to action being achieved through the Quintuple Helix paradigm and systemic concept of multi-actor engagement, knowledge sharing, production, and capital generation. The workstream works through sub-committees and aims to build local collaboration and co-creation of relevant actions through the establishment of Local Water Forums (LWF).

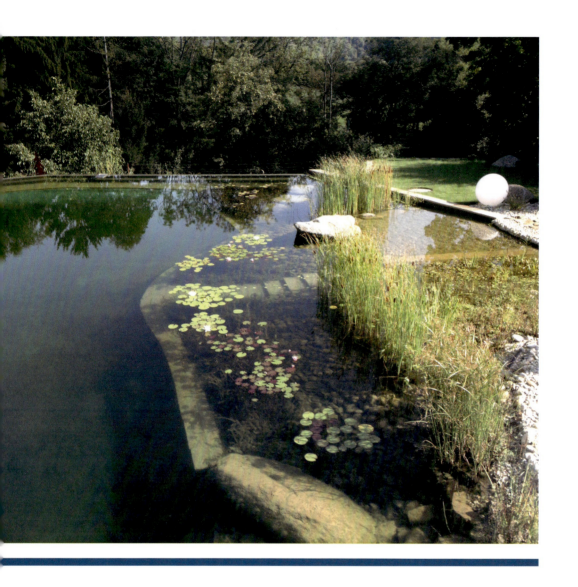

1 + 1 = 3 (AND EVEN MORE ...)

WATER STEWARDSHIP ACTION IN THE BEVERAGE INDUSTRY

Michael Dickstein (Sustainability/ESG Lead)

WATER STEWARDSHIP | AT THE HEART OF SDG 6

The private sector has a key responsibility to ensure the availability and sustainable management of 'clean water and sanitation for all', as set out in Sustainable Development Goal Number Six (SDG 6). Leading companies, particularly in the beverage sector, are gradually stepping up to protect and restore water-related ecosystems. Through innovative partnerships with the United Nations, NGOs, and local stakeholders, they launch initiatives to safeguard sustainable withdrawals and the supply of freshwater for their communities, and, in turn, for themselves.

Moreover, the current private sector trend towards net zero could have a positive impact on the sustainability of catchment areas, too.

WATER SCARCITY | AN INCREASING ISSUE FOR THE PRIVATE SECTOR

"The planet will survive no matter what. Life will continue with us or without us. What we have to do is save our species." © Simon Sinek[1]

As early as 1985, former UN Secretary General Boutros Boutros-Ghali warned that the next war in the Middle East would be fought over water, not politics. Sadly, the outbreak of the civil war in Syria ten years ago proved him right. The worst drought in 900 years had hit the country and forced rural populations to move to the cities looking for work. Tensions rose, leading to protests against the government and then straight to the armed conflict which still continues today.

At the latest since the war in Ukraine, there is widespread consensus about the geopolitical importance of the ESG2 agenda. The Grand Ethiopian Renaissance Dam on the Nile is the subject of ongoing controversy amid claims of rising water scarcity by Egypt, since the first of 13 turbines has started to generate electricity for Ethiopia last

---

1   Touchton, M. (2020) 'Simon Sinek Says We Got Global Warming Wrong' [Online]. Available at: https://medium.com/climate-conscious/simon-sinek-says-we-got-global-warming-wrong-22522b6d3484 (Accessed: 26 April 2022).

2   The author applies the acronym of Environmental, Social, and Corporate governance (ESG), which has gradually replaced the previous term of Corporate Social Responsibility (CSR) – all of which refer to the notion of sustainability in one way or the other.

February.3 Meanwhile, 32 water facilities in Burkina Faso have already been destroyed this year, impacting 300,000 civilians as part of a violent conflict.4

Current forecasts are grim. Without improvements in water management, the world will face a 40% shortfall between the forecasted demand and the available supply of water by 2030.5 Overall, scientists predict that a potential for drought-induced migration will increase by approximately 200 percent under the current international policy scenario (corresponding to the current Paris Agreement targets).6

Water availability is pivotal for our communities but also for a broad array of industries in the manufacturing process. From textiles and paper to chemicals and basic metals, water is required for fabricating, processing, washing, diluting, cooling, or transporting a product. Global companies are exposed to significant risks posed by depleted and contaminated water supplies; the potential value at risk tops out at a staggering US$225 billion.7

In particular, water is a central ingredient for the beverage sector, i.e. the single most essential ingredient in their products and a critical utility used throughout the supply chain. The lifeline of beverages literally depends on the continued availability of water for the next years and, actually, decades to come.

3   Schenk, A. (2022), 'Streit am Nil' [Online]. Available at https://www.zeit.de/2022/18/wasserversorgung-aegypten-aethiopien-nil?utm_referrer=https%3A%2F%2Fwww.bing.com%2F (Accessed on 03 May 2022).

4   Norwegian Refugee Council (2022) 'Burkina Faso: Over a quarter million people victims of new "water war" in peak dry season' [Online]. Available at: https://www.nrc.no/news/2022/may/burkina-faso-over-a-quarter-million-people-victims-of-new-water-war-in-peak-dry-season/ (Accessed: 03 May 2022).

5   The World Bank (2017), 'Water Resources Management' [Online]. Available at: https://www.worldbank.org/en/topic/waterresourcesmanagement#1 (Accessed: 26 April 2022).

6   Smirnov O. et al. (2022) 'Climate Change, Drought, and Potential Environmental Migration Flows Under Different Policy Scenarios' [Online]. Available at: https://journals.sagepub.com/doi/10.1177/01979183221079850 (Accessed: 09 May 2022).

7   Lamb C. et al. (2022) 'High and Dry. How Water Issues Are Stranding Assets' [Online]. Available at: https://cdn.cdp.net/cdp-production/cms/reports/documents/000/006/321/original/High_and_Dry_Report_Final.pdf?1651652748 (Accessed: 06 May 2022).

BUSINESS IMPERATIVE | THE CORPORATE APPROACH

The good news is that in recent years beverage companies have accelerated water stewardship activities in order to balance their own water use with the needs of communities and the environment. This industry trend emerged in the slipstream of a generic mindset shift towards ESG, i.e. from charities and philanthropic one-offs to a structured business imperative agenda. The new corporate adage is, that 'everything that we do in sustainability contributes either directly or indirectly to our key priorities'. As part of the risk mitigation process, initiatives are designed to enhance the resilience of own operations and the broader supply chain. Additionally, eco-efficiency projects are aimed at using less water (as well as energy, etc.). ESG even strives for new business opportunities, e.g. through sustainable product innovations or social marketing campaigns.

Global beverage leaders pursue their water stewardship agendas as they acknowledge the need for a 'social license to operate' in order to maintain and further grow their business. Corporate ESG strategies comprise of public commitments to reduce water consumption, to explore circular opportunities in catchment areas, and to safeguard the access to water and sanitation for local communities.

Some lead companies embarked on their water stewardship journey some 20 years ago when they started to bring the own house in order. They pursued water efficiency targets by reducing consumption levels, either absolutely or in relative terms, related to the volume of beverage produced. Gradually, such commitments became context-based, i.e. the focus on water stressed areas, e.g. in Southern Europe, parts of Africa, Latin America, or Asia. Simultaneously, the sector spent considerable investments to convert wastewater into an effluent that could be returned to the water cycle.

During the next phase, companies started to assess the future availability of water in their operations and to reduce related environmental and social risks. Today, source vulnerability assessments and related water protection plans are commonplace in the industry in order to assess the supply risk and to assure business continuity. Gradually, beverage producers are starting to work with suppliers on the water footprint of relevant (agricultural) raw materials. The most advanced businesses establish local and international partnership programmes to engage with communities for more awareness and protection of water resources. Global players also contribute to the development of water standards and policies in close cooperation with key stakeholders.

STAKEHOLDER ENGAGEMENT | FROM OBLIVION TO PARTNERSHIPS

Stakeholders have regularly ranked water availability among the top material issues for beverage producers. Conversely though, the industry had to learn the importance of the outreach to communities (and beyond) 'the hard way'.

Back in 2004, the Coca-Cola bottling company in India had to close a plant in the district of Kerala following major protests that erupted over allegations related to the water consumption. Local community groups had claimed that the catchment area was overly exploited, affecting farmlands in the area.[8] Apparently, Coca-Cola had not thought about the environmental implications when setting up their operations in Kerala; now they had to deal with the (financial and reputational) consequences.

Against the backdrop of this case, the industry had to course correct their approach. Beverage companies have launched various water stewardship initiatives with stakeholders, which do not form part of the group of 'usual suspects'. – Who would have thought that global brewers would partner with the United Nations for local projects in Ethiopia or Indonesia? That they would feature movie stars to raise awareness for water-carrying women in India? Or that soft drinks manufacturers would collaborate with global organisations and NGOs for restoration projects and access to freshwater? – Below are some industry examples:

In 2015, Heineken announced a strategic ESG partnership with the United Nations Industrial Development Organisation. The key objective was to deploy water stewardship initiatives in eleven regions classified as "water-scarce."[9] As a result, stakeholder workshops were launched in Ethiopia and Nigeria. In Indonesia, Heineken joined a water alliance comprising of government, NGOs, other businesses, and the local community. The aim is to reduce pollution in the Brantas river basin and to restore the watershed. In early 2022, an upscaling initiative was granted, co-funding for US1.8mln from the Global Environment Facility.[10]

8   For more information read 'Plachimada Coca-Cola struggle' [Online]. Available at https://en.wikipedia.org/wiki/Plachimada_Coca-Cola_struggle (Accessed: 26 April 2022).

9   Richie H. (2015) 'Heineken, UNIDO Team Up to Drive Sustainability Efforts in Water-Scarce Developing Markets' [Online]. Available at https://sustainablebrands.com/read/supply-chain/heineken-unido-team-up-to-drive-sustainability-efforts-in-water-scarce-developing-markets (Accessed: 26 April 2022).

10 Susan C. (2022), 'Maintaining and Enhancing Water Yield through Land & Forest Rehabilitation' [Online]. Available at https://open.unido.org/projects/ID/projects/200181 (Accessed: 26 April 2022).

Through the flagship brand Stella Artois, AB InBev has also engaged in water activities with water.org, a global nonprofit organisation focusing on water and sanitation. In a series of marketing campaigns with Matt Damon, a well-known actor, they promote access to clean water in India and other parts of the world. In a recent interview, Damon explained that through this partnership alone, the NGO had reached over three million people with safe water and sanitation in previous years.[11]

As the latest in a row of new corporate water stewardship ambitions, Procter & Gamble has announced to work with the World Resources Institute Water Programme to ensure the new water targets align with science-based requirements.[12] The overall aim is to restore more water than is lost in key regions where it operates.

In the meantime, Coca-Cola has accelerated their water stewardship agenda with various partnerships worldwide. They collaborate with the WWF to improve the health of freshwater basins and the environmental performance across Coca-Cola's supply chain, emissions, and packaging. As for Nigeria, they joined forces with the State Water Board and community groups in the Kano district, to progress a water supply project that will facilitate ground water exploration. Coca-Cola has installed flexible high-pressure pipes which transfer water from the Challawa River to the production plant. There it is sanitised to drinking quality for the community.[13] In 2020, Coca-Cola announced another initiative for effective water, sanitation, and hygiene services in Nigeria with the United States Agency for International Development as well as partnerships with other international aid organisations.[14]

Based on personal experience, successful cross-stakeholder partnerships showcase three key criteria, i.e.:
1. ***Create a level playing field***. By working together, partners must strive for a goal which reaches far beyond what could be achieved by working 'only' alongside each other.

---

11 Fitzgerald A. (2021) 'Matt Damon X Stella Artois Join Forces to Give Back' [Online]. Available at: https://www.forbes.com/sites/alissafitzgerald/2021/11/05/matt-damon-x-stella-artois-join-forces-to-give-back/?sh=7d9ecd8e69ae (Accessed: 27 April 2022).

12 Mace M. (2022) 'P&G to restore more water than used across key manufacturing locations' [Online]. Available at: https://www.edie.net/pg-to-restore-more-water-than-used-across-key-manufacturing-locations/ (Accessed: 20 June 2022).

13 'Water project in Challawa' [Online]. Available at https://www.coca-colahellenic.com/en/a-more-sustainable-future/performance/case-studies (Accessed: 26 April 2022).

14 Aliogo U. (2021) 'Nigeria: Coca-Cola System's Holistic Approach to Water Stewardship' [Online]. Available at: https://allafrica.com/stories/202111090086.html (Accessed: 26 April 2022).

2. ***Leave stereotypes behind***. NGOs are not just idealistic or unworldly philanthropists. In fact, they bring a lot of pragmatic, economic sense and experience to the table. In turn, corporations are not just a cash cow; they offer knowledge about markets, (consumer) behaviour, logistical questions, etc.

3. ***Allow for the relationship to evolve over time***. Cultural dispositions differ substantially from one business to the other, let alone between peculiar stakeholder groups. Partners should take their time for real mutual understanding. An open, candid, and transparent platform to address the issues of pace, processes, internal governance, mindset, and culture will facilitate that.

CLOSING THE LOOP | WATER-ENERGY-FOOD NEXUS

Sustainable water resources management is a key priority for the future of our planet or, to be more precise, for the future of mankind on this very planet. However, the climate debate and the worldwide quest to reduce emissions in recent years have seemingly overshadowed the importance of clean water and sanitation for all.

Lately, support for the water agenda is arising exactly from that angle. As part of the so-called nexus thinking, the complex interdependencies between water, energy, and food are unsurfacing. It will only be a matter of time before sectoral development interventions are going to be replaced by an integrated resource-use approach.

Amid the current wave of net zero commitments, companies realise that 100% of carbon emissions targets can only be achieved by a certain (limited) level of offsetting activities, i.e. to neutralise the impact of residual emissions that cannot be effectively eliminated through more energy efficiency or renewable sources. This conclusion offers an important link between climate action and water stewardship, as one key area for carbon offsetting relates to restoration (mostly, reforestation[15]) of rivers, wetlands, peat bogs, and other places for carbon sequestration.

Universities and other academic experts, along with the private sector, are currently exploring methods to quantify the impact of water-related initiatives in catchment areas for the carbon offsetting agenda. The results will form an additional boost for SDG 6 and the supply of freshwater for us all.

---

15 For an overview, see Bhatia V. (2022) 'Explainer: Carbon insetting vs offsetting' [Online]. Available at: https://www.weforum.org/agenda/2022/03/carbon-insetting-vs-offsetting-an-explainer/ (Accessed: 27 April 2022).

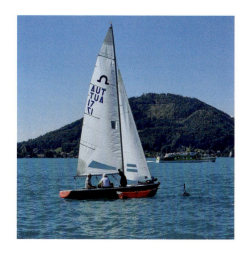
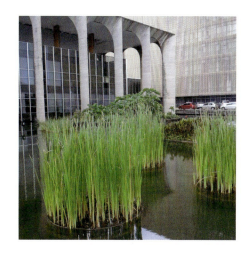
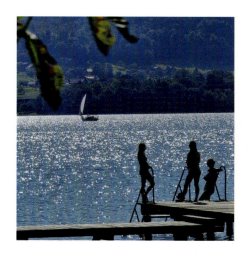
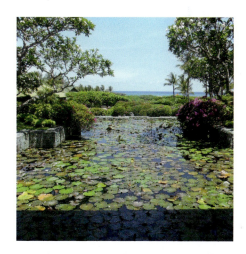
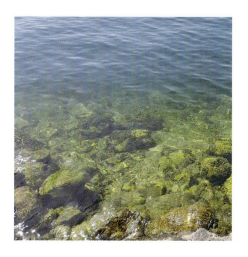
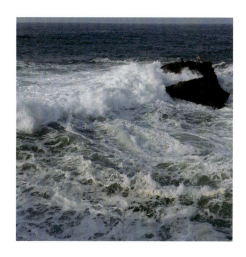

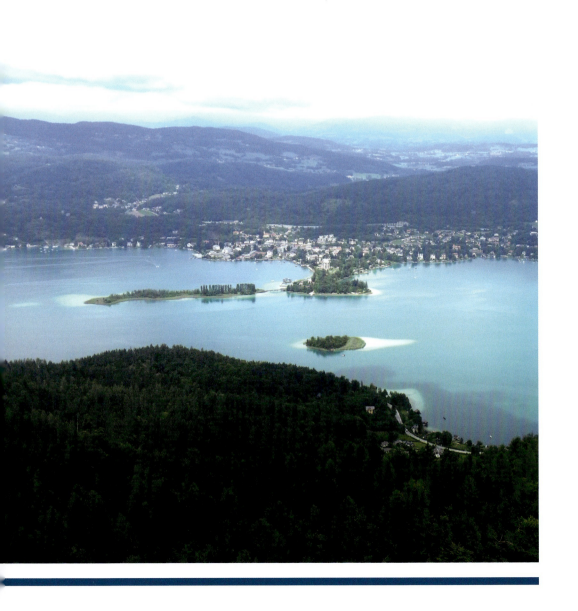

BUILDING EFFECTIVE WATER DIALOGUES AND ALLIANCES

MAKING INTERNATIONAL COOPERATION IN WATER INNOVATION WORK

Gaetano Casale et al. (IHE Delft Institute for Water Education)

Authors, co-authors, and contributors of the paper are core members of the Water Europe Working Group "Water Beyond Europe":

Gaetano Casale (Editor, IHE Delft Institute for Water Education); David Smith (Water, Environment and Business for Development); Dominique Darmendrail (BRGM), Lars Skov Andersen (China Resources Management), Ines Breda (Grundfos), Richard Elelman (EURECAT), Véronique Briquet-Laugier (ANR)

With contributions from:

Antonio Lo Porto (CNR IRSA); Paul Campling (VITO); Uta Wehn (IHE Delft); Diana Chavarro Rincon (ITC Enschede)

ABSTRACT

This article is built from the work of the Water Beyond Europe Working Group white paper. The article advocates that water, if not attended to in a manner beyond self-interest, will represent the biggest societal challenge of this century intertwined with the impacts of climate change. This article is also a contribution to recognise the significance of the SDG 17 ("Strengthen the means of implementation and revitalise the global partnership for sustainable development") as the overriding goal whose success will serve as a key enabler to accelerate the implementation of the SDG 6 ("Ensure availability and sustainable management of water and sanitation for all") in itself and in the broader context of the SDG agenda, as water resources are pivotal for many other SDGs. This calls for people to consciously agree to exploring the many values of water in different SDG settings. Furthermore, it is argued that the connection between SDG 6 and the remaining SDGs must first and foremost start with the human connection, embodied in SDG 17.

KEY MESSAGES

This article builds upon the main concepts included in global agendas and policies, such as the UN 2030 Agenda on Sustainable Development Goals (SDGs), the recommendations of the Intergovernmental Panel on Climate Change (IPCC), and the 1992 Dublin Statement on international water sector development. In such, the key messages derived from the Working Group are divided into 3 main areas: modalities; financing, and implementation.

Key Messages – on Modalities

Key Message 1: Cooperation on Water Beyond Europe is gradually shifting from top-down approaches to partnerships based on participatory approaches on an equal basis.

Key Message 2: Conscious stakeholder participation is imperative for sustainable development.

Key Messages – on Financing

Key Message 3: The eligibility for funding of international Research and Innovation (R&I) cooperation within the European Research Framework Programmes is crucial.

Key Message 4: The participation of the economic sector must be recognised and increased to achieve the SDGs and produce a significant societal impact.

Key Messages – on Implementation

Key Message 5: Pathways to impact is a long road that often stretches beyond individual programmes and projects.

Key Message 6: Living labs and knowledge hubs are important mechanisms where researchers and practitioners from industry, social, and natural sciences can work together in real life environments.

1. INTRODUCTION

This article addresses the modality and approach of the EU cooperation on Water Beyond Europe as a unique contribution to frame EU policies and actions within SDG17 "Strengthen the means of implementation and revitalise the global partnership for sustainable development," which is a prerequisite for the implementation of all other SDGs.

The target group of the white paper from the working group are policy makers, in particular members and staff of the European Parliament and Commission and of the European Member States, in charge of shaping the current and future EU international cooperation policies to support the effective and impactful implementation of EU supported R&I to solve global challenges. Furthermore, Water sector organisations need to support start-ups and the upscaling of their international cooperation efforts, in a way that supports a sustainable society.

The need for revitalised international cooperation has emerged in the past few decades as a new paradigm to bring forward innovative solutions, as global challenges are so interconnected and so huge that they cannot be addressed by single countries or sectors alone. They require an unprecedented level of mutual learning and cooperation amongst different actors with different perspectives across issues, sectors, and geographies.

Herein, we first discuss the global water challenges and make the case for more effective and impactful global partnership and cooperation; then we highlight best practices and shortcomings, based on which key recommendations for the strengthening of international cooperation are provided with the ultimate goal of delivering tangible on-the-ground contributions to the SDGs.

2. WATER AND THE SDGS

The Sustainable Development Goals, alongside the Intergovernmental Panel on Climate Change (IPCC), increasingly shape EU and global political agendas. SDG 6 is about water and is one of the most important SDGs as water is also a catalyst to achieve all of the remaining 16 SDGs1 as reflected in a number of recent EC policies2 3. The latest report from UN-Water highlights that SDG 6 is off-track, and therefore unprecedented actions are needed to accelerate SDG 6 achievement4. An important underlying factor is to ensure actions are better coordinated and that global cooperation and complementarity becomes the norm, hence the importance of giving more prominence to SDG 17 and its related targets as a means to achieve SDG 6 and other water related SDGs.

Water is also a key element in climate change. Its role in mitigation, prevention, and protection against climate change is significant on the global scale. According to the IPCC, 80% of climate change adaptation measures involve water5.

Science, Technology, and Innovation (STI) as well as building effective partnerships, and capacity development as cross-cutting processes, are clearly considered essential to achieve the SDGs and to highlight the importance of multi-stakeholder collaboration on STI for the SDGs between Member States, civil society, the economic sector, the scientific community, and United Nations entities. The importance of these aspects is also outlined in the EU Global Approach to Research and Innovation – EU strategy for

---

1   UN Water, Water and Sanitation Interlinkages across the 2030 Agenda for Sustainable Development [Online] Available at: https://www.unwater.org/publications/water-sanitation-interlinkages-across-2030-agenda-sustainable-development/

2   Council of the EU, EU Council Conclusions on Water Diplomacy 2021 [Online] Available at: https://www.consilium.europa.eu/en/press/press-releases/2021/11/19/water-in-diplomacy-council-confirms-eu-s-commitment-to-enhanced-eu-engagement/

3   Water and Beyond: Elements for a strategic approach on global and EU external action in the water sector 2021 [Online] Available at: https://op.europa.eu/en/publication-detail/-/publication/4c8df458-df93-11eb-895a-01aa75ed71a1/language-en

4   UN Water, The SDG 6 Global Acceleration Framework [Online] Available at: https://www.unwater.org/publications/the-sdg-6-global-acceleration-framework/

5   IPCC, Climate Change 2022: Impacts, Adaptation and Vulnerability [Online] Available at: https://www.ipcc.ch/report/sixth-assessment-report-working-group-ii/

international **cooperation in a changing world**[6] **as well as in the broader context of the EU Green Deal**[7].

3. THE GLOBAL WATER CHALLENGES

All of society's challenges, and therefore achievement of the SDGs, depend heavily on water – with water being mentioned explicitly or implicitly in each SDG. In particular, the role of SDG 17 as the **common enabling force is undervalued**. Attention to and recognition of SDG17, which includes the human dimension, effective cooperation, and working for a common good, needs to be increased.

When discussing water challenges, we have to realise that the benefits derived from water and the risks related to water are normally measured **from outside the water sector**, leading to a lack of accountability[8]. The significance of water is not sufficiently recognised at the political level, and therefore water challenges have not properly been addressed in R&I policies. In addition, international cooperation (closely related to SDG 17) as a standalone element is often taken for granted, vaguely "encouraged" but rarely specifically addressed, at the national or European levels to achieve enhanced long-term impact. Effective international cooperation creates a unique additional value for the achievement of the SDGs.[9]

Water is the leading component of the **Water-Energy-Food-Ecosystems-Health** Nexus (WEFEH) and those responsible for its management must establish a coherent permanent national and international dialogue with their partners in other sectors and furthermore take the lead in creating such initiatives, removing existing inter- and intra-sectoral fragmentation to ensure that global, social, and environmental issues are addressed correctly.

---

6   European Commission, Communication from the Commission to the European Parliament, the Council, the European Economic and Social Committee and the Committee of the Regions on the Global Approach to Research and Innovation [Online] Available at: https://eur-lex.europa.eu/legal-content/EN/TXT/?uri=COM:2021:252:FIN

7   European Commission, Communication from the Commission to the European Parliament, the European Council, the Council, the European Economic and Social Committee and the Committee of the Regions on the European Green Deal [Online] Available at: https://eur-lex.europa.eu/legal-content/EN/TXT/?qid=1576150542719&uri=COM%3A2019%3A640%3AFIN

8   Water Security for All paper (2019)

9   United Nations Department of Economic and Social Affairs (UNDESA), Maximizing the impact of partnerships for the SDGs: [online] available at: https://sustainabledevelopment.un.org/partnerships/guidebook UN World Water Development Report 2022: Groundwater, making the invisible visible (UN Water – UNESCO).

There is the potential that most water-related **health** effects could be adverse and could occur via direct exposures (for example, extreme weather events) and less direct influences arising from declining food yields, freshwater flows and quality, stability of infectious disease patterns, family incomes, and livelihoods.

Migration is associated with a) increased frequency of droughts that affect agricultural production, reducing livelihoods and access to clean water b) extreme weather events, such as frequent floods that destroy houses or arable land and force people to relocate, b) rising sea levels that render coastal areas uninhabitable, and d) competition over natural resources that may lead to conflict, which in turn exacerbates migration.[10]
Water has in many cases represented an almost sacred **transboundary** element. Rivers such as the Nile, the Danube, the Tigris, the Euphrates, or the Amazon that run across man-made borders have historically been immune to the effects of international rivalry and conflict, but unilateral upstream development is emerging, for example in the Middle East and North Africa (MENA) region.[11] This represents the perils of interregional and international **conflicts**, employed as a proactive, coercive arm (for example, the unspoken of ability of one state to obstruct the supply of water to another) whilst also passively becoming a victim of conflict.

The challenges that have been identified as a result of the COVID-19 pandemic have been illustrated even more clearly by the crisis in the Ukraine. The appalling consequences of the conflict demonstrate even more dramatically how local crisis can have effects globally and upon the interdependency of nation states around the world. The inability of Ukraine and Russia to export grain and seeds and the interruption of energy supplies have resulted in an immediate policy shift on the part of supranational agencies to concentrate their efforts on food and energy security. Water has a pivotal role to play in both contexts if widespread famine, energy poverty, and an increasingly unstable economic situation are to be addressed as both the World Bank[12] and the World Economic Forum have highlighted (the latter in all top global risks since 2015 as well as during the recent 2022 Davos Forum[13]).

---

10 Ebb and Flow, Volume 1: Water, Migration, and Development

11 SIWI World Water Week: Sowers, J. University of New Hamphire and the Crown Center for Middle Eastern Studies, Brandeis University

12 The Guardian, Ukraine war 'will mean high food and energy prices for three years' [Online] Available at: https://www. theguardian.com/business/2022/apr/26/ukraine-war-food-energy-prices-world-bank

13 World Economic Forum, Davos 2022 – What just happened? 9 things to know [Online] Available at: https://www. weforum.org/agenda/2022/05/the-story-of-davos-2022/?utm_source=sfmc&utm_medium=email&utm_ campaign=2778141_Agenda_weekly-27May2022&utm_term=&emailType=Agenda%20Weekly

The United Nations has made clear that "…one of the major challenges facing the world community as it seeks to replace unsustainable development patterns with environmentally sound and sustainable development is the need to activate a sense of common purpose on behalf of all sectors of society".[14] The probability of forging such a sense of purpose will depend on the willingness of all sectors to participate in genuine social partnership and dialogue, while recognising the independent roles, responsibilities, and special capacities of each party. Events such as the conflict in Ukraine demonstrate the need for a global reaction that underlines the importance of transboundary cooperation. From the tragic ashes of warfare, it is possible that a broader support for genuine cooperation across national divides in order to enhance sustainability emerges if action is rapidly initiated.[15]

4. OPPORTUNITIES GENERATED BY INTERNATIONAL R&I COOPERATION

Knowledge and Information

Awareness leads to concern, concern leads to engagement, engagement leads to social consensus, and social consensus leads to political continuity even on the international stage[16]. A new era of international enlightenment based on transparent and documented **information** is required to raise awareness among an ample, international, heterogeneous social audience with distinct levels of **technical comprehension** ranging from the concerned layman, students, to the professional stakeholder, the political decision-maker and the specialised scientific and technical expert.

The promoters of more efficient international water strategies and collaboration have at their disposal a wide range of exciting mechanisms to improve transparency and public perception, e.g. participatory science for data collection, Digital Social Platforms and Augmented Reality that are capable of demonstrating both financial and practical benefits in a clear and accessible manner thus activating a common sense of purpose. Wide-spread knowledge results in improved citizen engagement, and this will result in a **proactive involvement** in the co-creation, development, and subsequent implementation of international water policy.

---

14 United Nations Environment Programme Decision: 27.2.

15 Nature, What the war in Ukraine means for energy, climate and food [Online] Available at: https://www.nature.com/articles/d41586-022-00969-9

16 Elelman, R, Feldman, D.L. (2018) The future of citizen engagement in cities—The council of citizen engagement in sustainable urban strategies (ConCensus). Futures Volume 101, August 2018, Pages 80-91. https://doi.org/10.1016/j.futures.2018.06.012

Such practical communication and non-professional involvement results in a far broader social consensus on an international scale providing a far more solid base for policy continuity. The European Parliament, Commission, and the Member States of the European Union must act to ensure that all actors are trained in such social-oriented activities for their concrete implementation.[17]

Involvement of Concerned Stakeholders

Effective international water cooperation is based on the human element of **trust**. Trust is an essential and yet highly disregarded commodity. Trust, which is essential for any form of socio-political agreement, can only exist if a) all parties *are fully informed from the very outset* of an initiative of all the advantages and disadvantages and subsequent results of the action and b) if all social sectors within the affected communities are *truly engaged*.

There is a need to activate a sense of **common purpose** on behalf of all sectors of society. Both the bottom-up and top-down approaches must be adhered to in order to acquire the necessary global and societal consensus that will guarantee effective intra- and supra-national policy continuity, implemented in local communities. The probability of forging such a sense of purpose depends on the willingness of all sectors to participate in genuine social partnership and dialogue while recognising the independent roles, responsibilities, and special capacities of each.[18]

5. INTERNATIONAL COOPERATION SUPPORTING WATER INNOVATION

International cooperation is required to tackle the global water challenges expressed in the SDGs and their global connections. Across the globe, joint transnational activities should be carried out to address the major societal challenges and to create value and jobs. SDG 17 calls for enhanced global cooperation on issues like science, technology, innovation, and capacity development, placing them at the core of sustainable development.

---

17 Further references:
United Nations Environment Program (UNEP). Livelihood Security: Climate Change, Migration and Conflict in the Sahel. [Online] Available at: http://www.unep.org/pdf/UNEP_Sahel_EN.pdf (accessed on 22 March 2021).
Human Tide: The Real Migration Crisis. [Online] Available at: https://www.christianaid.org.uk/Images/human-tide.pdf (accessed on 12 March 2021).
Werz, M. and Hoffmann, M. (2016) Europe's twenty-first century challenge: climate change, migration and security. European View (2016) 15:145–154 DOI 10.1007/s12290-016-0385-7

18 Chen, A., Elelman, R. et al. (2021) The need for digital water in a green Europe [Online] Available at: https://op.europa.eu/en/publication-detail/-/publication/f68e3f26-821a-11eb-9ac9-01aa75ed71a1/language-en/format-PDF/source-search#

However, both regional and national interests based on political party interest, and racial, religious, and national bias are obstacles that constitute bottlenecks to international collaboration. Realistic pathways must be established that **enable supranational strategies to be converted into local action.** Municipal as well as rural concerns must be heard in the European Parliament and Commission and the United Nations Environment Assembly. The work, for example, of the United Nations World Water Quality Alliance Social Engagement Platform, coordinated by UNEP, is based on this philosophy. By creating Local Water Fora,19 the administrations responsible for the achievement of the ambitions of SDG 6 are turning to local communities to act as their representatives whilst establishing a pathway to international collaboration, which would be unthinkable, if responsibility were to lay on the shoulders of national governments.

Engagement Mechanisms

The general underlying principle of effective engagement is that, when relevant, stakeholders at local, regional, national, and international levels participate in a transparent process of co-creation, implementation, and post-implementation review of a broad range of water-based policies that reflect their needs and visions in the authority, enterprise, and research domains, as well as the perspectives of the civil society and the natural environment.[20] [21]

There are five principal engagement mechanisms which can be established and coordinated in order to achieve the ambitions of both supranational and locally based entities, which in turn act in perfect alignment with the EU Green Deal[22] and meet the UN intentions:

1. **True inter-sectoral nexus collaboration approach** between all sectors of a sustainable community: water, energy, food, waste, transport, health, social services, employment, etc.
2. **Supranational strategies including sustainability aspects** must be implemented by regional and local stakeholders in order to ensure the viability of long-term awareness creation, policy co-creation, and political continuity.

---

19 UNEP, World Water Quality Alliance, [Online] Available at: https://communities.unep.org/display/WWQA

20 The 1992 Dublin Statement

21 European Commission, Digital single market [Online] Available at: https://ec.europa.eu/digital-single-market/en/open-innovation-20

22 European Commission, A European Green Deal striving to be the first climate-neutral continent [Online] Available at: https://ec.europa.eu/info/strategy/priorities-2019-2024/european-green-deal_en

3. The **Quintuple Innovation Helix** i.e. the public authorities' sector, economic sector, research sector, citizens, and representatives of socio-cultural entities (in which knowledge is the main constituent), and must be involved at all stages of policy creation and the resulting implementation.

4. **The incorporation of new knowledge or innovation and their dissemination to local schools, colleges, and universities** is also of great significance as is a general approach to youth.

5. There needs to be a **greater understanding of the connections between the different organisations / institutions**, which have the influence, the networking ability, and the power to lead within the different networks and communities.

6. **Communication and knowledge exchange** should target municipalities, regions, and river basin authorities, as well as the economic sector. This will entail, among other actions, the establishment of an open-source Best Practice Repository (BPR), making the objectives and actions of international organisations accessible to all social sectors and all age-groups no matter their geographical location.

Special attention should be paid to the use and definition of the concept of participation to keep it meaningful in policy frameworks, where it can cover a wide range of experiences and different degrees of stakeholder engagement (e.g. the participatory ladder of consultation, partnership, delegated power, citizen control).

6. FUNDING R&I DEVELOPMENT AND IMPLEMENTATION

To broaden international cooperation in R&I on water challenges, specific instruments and mutual understandings have been built during the past few decades. International Cooperation for R&I is funded through different mechanisms depending on the activity and the recipient country's economy status.

- **For countries with low incomes** collaborating with European partners can be challenging. Development aid programmes focussing on joint collaboration can be a solution, even if they do not target R&I. The new EC DG International Partnership (DG-INTPA)[23] (former DG Development Cooperation) is opening funding schemes that compensate the lack of funds of the low-income country. The EU R&I framework programmes allow participation of legal entities from associated countries under equivalent conditions as legal entities from the EU Member States, unless specific limitations or conditions are laid down in the work programme. Participants from many low- to middle-income countries are automatically eligible for funding.

---

23 DG INTPA, International partnerships [Online] Available at: International Partnerships | European Commission (europa.eu)

- **For countries in transition from low to middle income status** development cooperation will shift from development aid to peer-to-peer partnerships as a more appropriate mechanism to maintain mutually beneficial existing cooperation based on earlier capacity-building efforts. This has been applied to water policy support and R&I funding at the EU level: the EC has developed "bilateral programmes" for water with, for example India[24] and China[25], in which these countries are directly supporting research and innovation contributors in their respective countries.
- **Funding mechanisms in a win-win manner, in which all countries participate in the funding**: The most typical instrument is a call for proposals with a virtual common pot. All participating countries enter a Memorandum of Understanding with a certain budget to fund the research groups of their country. An excellent example is the Horizon Europe partnership Water4All, which is open to EU Member States and beyond EU partners (e.g. Israel, Moldova, or South Africa).
- **Specific instruments** have also been developed to ease the participation of less experienced countries in R&I programmes:
  - *Thematic Annual Programming (TAP) Action for a common research priority.* The TAP Action gathers a cluster of R&I projects selected from recently funded projects at the national level or selected after the launch of a common call text agreed by funders.
  - *Knowledge hub (KH), for knowledge sharing, transfer, and dissemination* is a network of selected researchers within a defined scientific area and involved in R&I projects funded within the umbrella of the Water JPI[26] or at the national level.
  - *Living labs* is an essential approach which enables co-design, co-creation, and taking R&I from research to practice by demonstrating new technologies or innovative approaches by partners within and beyond Europe.

Financing international cooperation in the modalities mentioned above is undertaken through a number of different institutions and instruments, among others:
- Global cooperation with the European Research and Innovation Framework Programmes (currently Horizon Europe)
- Multilateral country cooperation (co-development and equal-footing cooperation in JPI or Partnerships)

---

24 India EU Water Partnership, Homepage [Online] Available at: IEWP | India-EU Water Partnership

25 China Europe Water Platform, Homepage [Online] Available at: Home | CEWP

26 Seven calls up to date have been launched under the Water JPI (Joint Programming Initiative) scheme, www.waterjpi.eu.

- Bilateral country cooperation, by the European Commission (INTPA) or individual Member States (development aid, research support)
- Large Enterprise Foundations (e.g. Veolia, Danone, Grundfos)
- Charities (e.g. Bill and Melinda Gates Foundation)
- Investment funds and International Financing Institutions (e.g. European Investment Bank and Nordic Investment Bank).

In conclusion, there are a number of financial arrangements available to support water research, innovation, and demonstration. However, these schemes are very dynamic and need to be closely monitored as more funding players and instruments might become available on the global scale. In addition, **insufficient attention in the funding arena is being paid to SDG17 when discussing water related challenges, and in the future, specific financial support to (new forms of) international cooperation and to the capacity to innovate might bring unprecedented results.**

7. FINDINGS AND RECOMMENDATIONS

In this paper, we have discussed the potential of achieving the SDG 17 as the main instrument to address all water related SDGs. We demonstrated the importance and gravity of water challenges as well as the opportunities that especially research, knowledge transfer, and international cooperation address, as well as the key aspect of financing international cooperation.

SDG 17 in all its different aspects of resource mobilisation (domestic, European, and international), multiple source financing and investment, policy coherence, and increased cooperation on key aspects like Science, Technology, Innovation and capacity development, is essential to achieve the SDG 6 and other connected SDGs of the 2030 agenda.

The main findings and recommendations suggesting a way forward can be summarised as follows.

- **All current funding mechanisms are necessary as major global societal challenges cannot be addressed individually** by each country or funder, consistently with the main messages of SDG 17 and in particular its targets related to resource mobilisation. In particular, the complementarity of the funding mechanisms is a strong added value to tackle global water challenges.
- In global cooperation, **the eligibility for funding within the European Framework Programmes is crucial.** Several external countries have been eligible for funding throughout the EU R&I Framework Programmes. Consequently, the European Union supports activities in priority areas specific to each country to promote cooperation in

all dimensions in water resources management. The balanced multilateral cooperation, such as the model developed by the Water JPI for the past ten years, seems to offer more benefits[27], i.e. co-development of strategic research and innovation agenda and implementation tools, increased participation of funding organisations in joint calls, increased number of R&I development teams in funded projects, diversity and relevance of joint actions.

- **The participation of the economic sector must be encouraged and increased to reach the global goals and to produce a significant societal impact.** Consequently, the R&I needs and capacity of the economic sector must be considered as soon as possible, and include private entities, small, medium and large enterprises in the strategic agendas setting. The **choice of thematic priorities and the targeted areas** worldwide should be the incentive to have the economic sector join the funding of R&I projects, based on the demand driven and not supply driven approaches.

- **Facilitate co-design and co-creation**: involving local / regional partners and business from the very start and during the whole project cycle is necessary and important to fill the gap between the cultural differences.

- **Promote living labs and knowledge hubs where researchers** from enterprises, social and natural sciences **work together in the real life environment with relevant end-users**. These tools allow targeted interventions with a cross-sector nexus approach.

- **Increase flexibility of cooperation modes to increase the number of joint activities across countries**: EU or non-EU countries have different national eligibility criteria that can hamper the launching of joint activities. More **alignment of rules and practices** is required to increase impacts.

- **Support a long-term engagement** to ensure proper outcomes and prevent adverse stop-and-go effects and waste of resources.

- **Calls for R&I projects** are still very important means for starting up and strengthening international cooperation, especially in relation to proposals that are based on existing projects and/or proposals that support existing networks and alliances.

- **Pathways to Impact is a long road**: Measuring research impact is of critical importance to research funders interested in ensuring that the research they fund is both scientifically excellent and has a meaningful impact on the grand challenges they are targeting and other outcomes.
  Nevertheless, demonstrating and communicating value from the research is complicated by many factors.[28]

---

27 cf. ERALEARN Workshop on globalization, April 2021

28 Darmendrail D, Wemaere A. (2021) Water Research and Innovation Partnership addressing Sustainable Development Goals, In: Leal Filho W., Azul A.M., Brandli L., Lange Salvia A., Wall T. (eds) Clean Water and Sanitation. Encyclopedia of the UN Sustainable Development Goals. Springer, Cham. DOI : 10.1007/978-3-319-70061-8_124-1

- **Building Linkages Research and related Aid Capacities for Developing Countries**: some networks have established strong linkages that also support the development of capacity to conduct research with countries beyond Europe. For example, the Water JPI established close linkages with South Africa (first non-European country to join the Water JPI).
- **Focus on engagement of civil society**: Engagement must extend to all social sectors. Neither race nor religion, economic status nor social class, gender nor age should be a constraint on participation. Qualification for involvement rather than membership in professional networks should be the interest and concern of the participant.
- **Encourage the use of brokers**, between capital investors, enterprises, policymakers, and research institutions to better connect the multiple parties involved. Money itself is not the **main problem, more important are the incentives** to conduct water R&I by different stakeholders, each one having their own interest to participate.
- **Diversity factor**: doors should be more open to next generation, considering not only culture and gender but also age as a diversity factor. A cultural and gender diverse youth representation in decision making positions (steering groups and boards) is required to discuss the values of water, based on an updated understanding of the water crises and access to the latest knowledge. The **intergenerational engagement (that can be accelerated by the next generation's familiarity with social platforms) enables a novel way to discuss water**, creating committed relationships between the leaders of today and the leaders of tomorrow, meaning continuous engagement based on an honest conversation about water values and the construction of a conscious strategic response to the water crises.

We support the promotion of the above-mentioned findings and recommendations and are committed to advocate the importance of the messages in the remainder of the UN 2030 Agenda for Sustainable Development, for example in the process leading to the UN Water Conference in 2023, a milestone event and the second ever UN Conference on Water after the first UN Water Conference held in Mar del Plata (Argentina) in 1977.

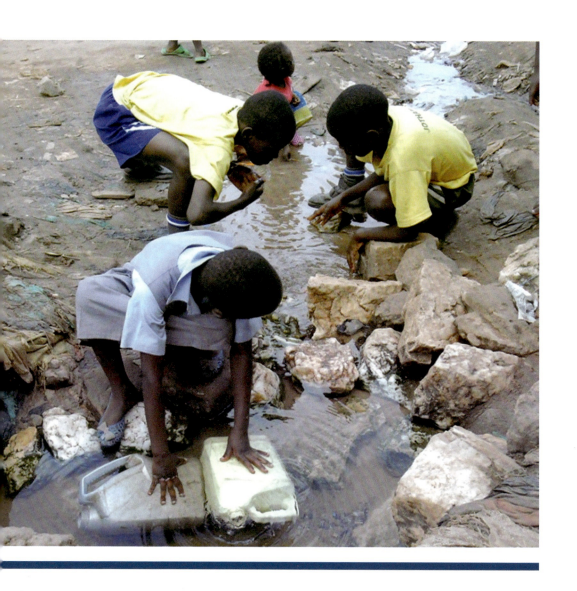

INTEGRATED APPROACHES AND STRATEGIES TO ADDRESS THE SANITATION CRISIS IN UNSEWERED SLUM AREAS IN AFRICAN MEGA-CITIES

Jan Willem Foppen (IHE Delft),
Piet N.L. Lens (National University Ireland, Galway)

SANITATION IN URBAN SLUMS OF DEVELOPING COUNTRIES

The rates of urbanisation and urban slum growth in developing countries – especially in sub-Saharan Africa, South America, and Asia – are estimated to be increasing and higher than the rate of urban infrastructure, and services provision (Isunju et al., 2011). Urban slums are characterised by high population density, population dynamics, poor urban infrastructure and lack of legal status (Katukiza et al., 2010). These factors make the provision of sustainable sanitation services difficult, which has also led to the increase of an urban population without access to improved sanitation in major urban centres in developing countries (Cairncross, 2006). In addition, the funds budgeted for the water and sanitation sector, for example, are mainly spent on water supply infrastructure, which has further weakened the sanitation sub-sector leading to the sanitation targets not being met by most developing countries (Joyce et al., 2010).

Generally, the inadequate collection and treatment of the waste streams (excreta, grey water, and solid waste) and the safe disposal or reuse of the end products are a threat to the environment and a risk to public health. In urban slums, soil and water sources (such as boreholes, shallow wells, springs, and streams) are contaminated with pathogens (bacteria and viruses), nutrients (nitrate, NO_3^-; ammonium, NH_4^+ and phosphate, PO_4^{3-}), and micro-pollutants (Katukiza et al., 2013; Nyenje et al., 2013). In particular pit latrines in slums contaminate ground water sources (Graham and Polizzotto, 2013; Nyenje et al., 2013), which may have negative health impacts on the slum dwellers. Moreover, high child mortality rates and loss of working days as a result of morbidity in urban poor areas are attributed to inadequate sanitation and poor hygienic practices (Genser et al., 2008). Provision of adequate and improved sanitation in slums is thus driven by the need to improve the quality of life by protecting the exposed population from infectious diseases, to reduce the deterioration of water sources, to protect the ecosystem downstream from the urban slums, and to recover waste for economic benefits in the form of renewable energy, reclaimed water, and recyclable solid materials (Katukiza et al., 2012).

CASE STUDY IN SLUM BWAISE III (KAMPALA, UGANDA)

A study was carried out in the framework of the interdisciplinary research project *Sanitation Crisis in Unsewered Slum Areas in African Mega-cities* (SCUSA). The aim of the SCUSA project was to contribute to sanitation improvement in urban slums by integrating the technical, socio-economic, and hydrological aspects of sanitation in slums. The study area of the SCUSA project was Bwaise III in Kampala, Uganda (Figure 1).

The specific objectives of this study:

- To assess the sanitation situation in the urban slum of Bwaise III in Kampala (Uganda) and to develop a method for the selection of sustainable sanitation technologies.
- To provide an insight into the magnitude of microbial risks to public health caused by pathogens through various exposure pathways in typical urban slums, such as Bwaise III in Kampala (Uganda).
- To design, implement, and evaluate the performance of a grey water treatment technology (prototype) in an urban slum.

GROUNDWATER POLLUTION IN UNSEWERED SLUMS

The majority of sanitation facilities in the slum are the so-called raised pit latrines (Figure 1b). They are raised, since the largest part of the pit below the superstructure is above the ground surface in order to avoid contact with the very shallow groundwater (10-50 cm below the surface). The effect of faecal sludge in the cesspits was assessed, both below and above the ground. Underground, in the shallow aquifer, a significant pollution to groundwater originating from pit latrines was found. However, it was estimated that approximately 2-20% of total N and less than 1% of total P mass input was lost to groundwater from the pit latrines (Nyenje et al., 2013). This indicates that in Bwaise III, pit latrines were very effective for the removal of nutrients.

In a next step, throughout the Bwaise III slum, groundwater observation wells were installed to study groundwater flow and groundwater quality. Groundwater appeared to be highly mineralised with high EC values, high Cl- concentrations, and high alkalinity concentrations. Furthermore, ammonium (NH_4^+) was the dominant N-species, while, to our surprise, ortho-phosphate ($o-PO_4^{3-}$) was generally absent. The plume of contaminants originated from wastewater leachates from pit latrines. Distinct redox zones in the direction of ground water flow were observed, which changed from nitrate-reducing upstream from Bwaise III to strongly iron (Fe) reducing downstream from Bwaise III. These redox changes were attributed to both the high residence times of groundwater of around 20 years, while on the other hand, the continuous degradation of mobile organic matter originating from the cesspools was held responsible for the greatly reducing conditions in the shallow aquifer. This suggests that lateritic alluvial sand aquifers are an effective sink of sanitation-related nutrients due to strong Fe-reducing conditions that favoured N removal by denitrification and PO_4^{3-} removal by chemical precipitation.

QUANTITATIVE MICROBIAL RISK ASSESSMENT

Realising that most of the surface waters in the area are diluted grey water mixed with some faecal sludge, the pathogenic viral load in various surface waters, groundwaters, and springs used for drinking water was determined (Katukiza et al., 2013; 2015). Our results indicated that various pathogenic viruses (rotavirus, adenovirus, and hepatitis A) were present in the slum environment and that their concentrations were rather high. With these data, a quantitative microbial risk assessment (QMRA) was carried out as an alternative approach for prioritising sanitation interventions (Katukiza et al., 2013). We found that the total disease burden was 9,549 disability-adjusted life years (DALYs) per year. The highest disease burden was 5,043 DALYs per year from exposure to bacteria and viruses in open drainage channels, which was 53% of the total disease burden. Please note that these results showed that the disease burden from all exposure routes was much higher than the WHO tolerable risk of 0.000001 DALYs per person per year (Cookey et al., 2016).

FAECAL SLUDGE

Above ground, we looked at how cesspits were emptied. We found that individual private cesspool operators or the Kampala City Council Authority (KCCA) were either too expensive for slum dwellers or simply could not access the slum. Through interviewing slum dwellers, we established the presence of a vivid manual emptying industry, which provided services for less than half of the price of the cesspool emptying trucks. These manual emptiers dispose of the faecal sludge originating from cesspits into a nearby drainage channel – a pit, which is dug besides the cesspit to be emptied – or simply on 'open ground'. Of course, each disposal method has its price. Because of the poor disposal practices (Figure 1d), manual emptying services are considered illegal. So, while emptying, they were always on the look-out for health inspectors and/or local council leaders to avoid being arrested for improper sludge disposal. This kind of working environment did not give them room to deliver their services effectively.

In the slum, faecal sludge has no added value. Not for slum dwellers, not for manual emptiers, and not for truck emptiers. However, we are convinced that a change in this attitude is part of the solution. That is, in relation to achieving a reduction of nutrients discharging the slum but likely also in relation to achieving a healthier slum environment. The conversion of organic waste or faecal sludge via the process of hydrothermal carbonisation (HTC), also known as wet coalification (Chung et al., 2014), leads to a black carbon type of product, which, when added to simple sand columns, is able to remove large quantities of the toxic metal ions cadmium (Minani et al., 2014), copper (Spataru et al., 2016) and arsenic (Wongrod et al., 2019). Also, HTC is able to drastically reduce the presence of *Escherichia coli* (Chung et al., 2017) as well as rotavirus and adenovirus (Chung et al., 2015; 2016) concentrations in water, which were passed through columns composed of HTC mixed with sand in set-ups in the laboratory.

Although more research has to be done, HTC is a good example of adding value to faecal sludge (Figure 3). The caloric value of faecal sludge harvested from cesspits in slums is higher than that of coffee husks used to fuel ovens for the tile baking industry (Muspratt et al., 2014). Alternatively, dried faecal sludge can be used for the production of tiles (Muspratt et al., 2014). This is another example of the conversion of faecal sludge into a valuable commodity, which is able to make one or more locally popular industrial process more efficient and/or cheaper.

GREY WATER

At least 50% of the surface water in Bwaise is grey water, originating from the kitchen, from washing clothes, or from the bathroom with very high nitrogen and phosphorus loads (Katikuza et al. 2013; 2015). Only a fraction of these concentrations is required to cause eutrophication. We estimated the grey-water volume discharging the slum to be around 200-300 mm annually, which was in the same range as the annual precipitation excess (precipitation minus evapotranspiration) of around 300 mm.

Realising the importance of grey water, a grey water filter was constructed with the main aim of reducing pollution. Thereto, various set-ups using locally available and cheap filter materials were tested in the laboratory of Makerere University (Katikuza et al., 2014b; 2014c). Then, a two-step crushed lava rock filter unit was designed and implemented for use by a household in the Bwaise III slum in Kampala (Figure 4). Katikuza et al. (2014c) reached removal efficiencies of chemical oxygen demand (COD), total phosphorous (TP), and Total Kjeldahl Nitrogen (TKN) of 91%, 60%, and 69%, respectively. The log removal of *E. coli*, *Salmonella* spp., and total coliforms were 3.9, 3.5, and 3.9, respectively. These results indicated that the use of the 2-step filter was a success, and functioned according to what it was originally designed for in the laboratory.

RECOMMENDATIONS FOR INTERVENTIONS

Based on our work in the Bwaise III slum, a number of ways forward which aim to reduce pollution downstream in the catchment in a cheap and sustainable way can be proposed:
- To actively treat grey water originating from households.
- The manual emptying organisations are key in preventing pollution of faecal matter in drains, especially since they are the ones emptying cesspits by disposing of faecal sludge into the drains. Legalising their work while at the same time facilitating the

connection between manual emptiers and private or public truck emptying services seem to be important ingredients in pollution prevention. At the same time, we hypothesise that an active channel clean keeping program, carried out by public entities, like the KCCA, in order to keep the channels free from solid waste, could assist in reducing pollution in drains originating from faecal matter.

- To convert faecal sludge into a valuable commodity which is able to make one or more locally popular industrial processes more efficient and/or cheaper. This will prevent the wasteful disposal of faecal sludge into drains, and can therefore not only make industrial processes cheaper, but it also prevents the pollution of surface waters downstream from the slum in the catchment.

ACKNOWLEDGEMENTS

This research has been carried as part of the research that was funded by the Netherlands Ministry of Development Cooperation (DGIS) through the UNESCO-IHE Partnership Research Fund. It was carried out jointly with UNESCO-IHE, Makerere University, and the Kampala City Council in the framework of the Research Project 'Addressing the Sanitation Crisis in Unsewered Slum Areas of African Mega-cities' (SCUSA). Project details have been communicated via the website *scusa.un-ihe.org*. Within the SCUSA project, Alex Katukiza made the PhD thesis *Sanitation in unsewered urban poor areas: Technology selection, quantitative microbial risk assessment and grey water treatment*. This chapter has not been subjected to peer and/or policy review by the DGIS, and, therefore, does not necessarily reflect the view of the DGIS.

REFERENCES

Cairncross S., 2006. Sanitation and water supply: practical lessons from the decade. UNDP – World Bank Water and Sanitation Program, The International Bank for Reconstruction and Development/The World Bank, Washington, D.C.

Chung, J. W., J. W. Foppen, M. Izquierdo & P. N. L. Lens, 2014. Removal of *Escherichia coli* from saturated sand columns supplemented with hydrochar produced from maize. Journal of Environmental Quality 43(6):2096-2103 doi:10.2134/jeq2014.05.0199.

Chung, J. W., J. W. Foppen, G. Gerner, R. Krebs & P. N. L. Lens, 2015. Removal of rotavirus and adenovirus from artificial ground water using hydrochar derived from sewage sludge. Journal of Applied Microbiology 119(3):876-884 doi:10.1111/jam.12863.

Chung, J. W., M. Breulmann, A. Clemens, C. Führer, J. W. Foppen & P. N. L. Lens, 2016. Simultaneous removal of rotavirus and adenovirus from artificial ground water using hydrochar derived from swine feces. Journal of Water and Health 14(5):754-767 doi:10.2166/wh.2016.010.

Chung, J. W., O. C. Edewi, J. W. Foppen, G. Gerner, R. Krebs & P. N. L. Lens, 2017. Removal of *Escherichia coli* by intermittent operation of saturated sand columns supplemented with hydrochar derived from sewage sludge. Applied Sciences (Switzerland) 7(8) doi:10.3390/app7080839.

Cookey, P. E., T. Koottatep, P. van der Steen & P. N. L. Lens, 2016. Public health risk assessment tool: Strategy to improve public policy framework for onsite wastewater treatment systems (OWTS). Journal of Water Sanitation and Hygiene for Development 6(1):74-88 doi:10.2166/washdev.2016.081.

Genser, B., Strina, A., dos Santos, L.A., Teles, C.A., Prado, M.S., Cairncross, S., Barreto, M.L., 2008. Impact of a city-wide sanitation intervention in a large urban centre on social, environmental and behavioural determinants of childhood diarrhoea: analysis of two cohort studies. International Journal of Epidemiology 37(4), 831 -840.

Graham. J.P., Polizzotto, M.L., 2013. Pit latrines and their impacts on groundwater quality: a systematic review. Environmental Health Perspectives 121(5), 521-30.

Isunju, J.B., Schwartz, K., Schouten, M.A., Johnson, W.P., van Dijk, M.P., 2011. Socioeconomic aspects of improved sanitation in slums: A review. Public Health 125, 368-376.

Joyce, J., Granit, J., Frot, E., Hall, D., Haarmeyer, D., Lindström A., 2010. The Impact of the Global Financial Crisis on Financial Flows to the Water Sector in Sub-Saharan Africa. Stockholm, SIWI.

Katukiza, A. Y., M. Ronteltap, A. Oleja, C. B. Niwagaba, F. Kansiime & P. N. L. Lens, 2010. Selection of sustainable sanitation technologies for urban slums – A case of Bwaise III in Kampala, Uganda. Science of the Total Environment 409(1):52-62 doi:10.1016/j.scitotenv.2010.09.032.

Katukiza, A. Y., M. Ronteltap, C. B. Niwagaba, J. W. A. Foppen, F. Kansiime & P. N. L. Lens, 2012. Sustainable sanitation technology options for urban slums. Biotechnology Advances 30(5):964-978 doi:10.1016/j.biotechadv.2012.02.007.

Katukiza, A. Y., H. Temanu, J. W. Chung, J. W. A. Foppen & P. N. L. Lens, 2013. Genomic copy concentrations of selected waterborne viruses in a slum environment in Kampala, Uganda. Journal of Water and Health 11(2):358-370 doi:10.2166/wh.2013.184.

Katukiza, A. Y., M. Ronteltap, C. B. Niwagaba, F. Kansiime & P. N. L. Lens, 2014a. Grey water treatment in urban slums by a filtration system: Optimisation of the filtration medium. Journal of Environmental Management 146:131-141 doi:10.1016/j.jenvman.2014.07.033.

Katukiza, A. Y., M. Ronteltap, C. B. Niwagaba, F. Kansiime & P. N. L. Lens, 2014b. A two-step crushed lava rock filter unit for grey water treatment at household level in an urban slum. Journal of Environmental Management 133:258-267 doi:10.1016/j.jenvman.2013.12.003.

Katukiza, A. Y., M. Ronteltap, P. van der Steen, J. W. A. Foppen & P. N. L. Lens, 2014c. Quantification of microbial risks to human health caused by waterborne viruses and bacteria in an urban slum. Journal of Applied Microbiology 116(2):447-463 doi:10.1111/jam.12368.

Katukiza, A. Y., M. Ronteltap, C. B. Niwagaba, F. Kansiime & P. N. L. Lens, 2015. Grey water characterisation and pollutant loads in an urban slum. International Journal of Environmental Science and Technology 12(2):423-436 doi:10.1007/s13762-013-0451-5.

Minani, J. M. V., J. W. Foppen & P. N. L. Lens, 2014. Sorption of cadmium in columns of sand-supported hydrothermally carbonized particles. Water Science and Technology 69(12):2504-2509 doi:10.2166/wst.2014.175.

Muspratt, A.M., Nakato, T., Niwagaba, C., Dione, H., Kang, J., Stupin, L., Regulinski, J., Mbéguéré, M., Strande, L. 2014. Fuel potential of faecal sludge: Calorific value results from Uganda, Ghana and Senegal. Journal of Water Sanitation and Hygiene for Development 4(2), 223-230. Doi: 10.2166/washdev.2013.055.

Nyenje, P.M., Foppen, J.W., Kulabako, R., Muwanga, A., Uhlenbrook, S., 2013. Nutrient pollution in shallow aquifers underlying pit latrines and domestic solid waste dumps in urban slums. Journal of Environmental Management 122, 15-24.

Spataru, A., R. Jain, J. W. Chung, G. Gerner, R. Krebs & P. N. L. Lens, 2016. Enhanced adsorption of orthophosphate and copper onto hydrochar derived from sewage sludge by KOH activation. RSC Advances 6(104):101827-101834 doi:10.1039/c6ra22327c.

Wongrod, S., S. Simon, E. D. van Hullebusch, P. N. L. Lens & G. Guibaud, 2019. Assessing arsenic redox state evolution in solution and solid phase during As(III) sorption onto chemically-treated sewage sludge digestate biochars. Bioresource Technology 275:232-238 doi:10.1016/j.biortech.2018.12.056.

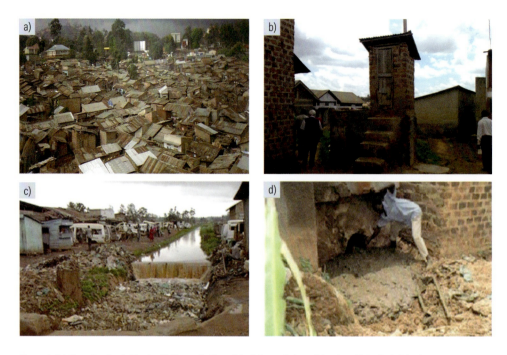

Figure 1. Existing situation in Bwaise III (Kampala, Uganda). a) General view of the slum, b) Typical pit latrine, c) Water channel for drainage blocked by solid waste, and d) Typical manual cesspit emptying

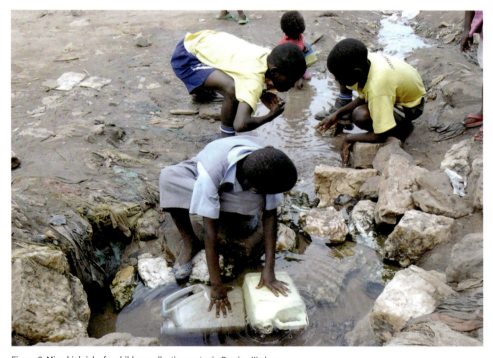

Figure 2. Microbial risks for children collecting water in Bwaise III slum.

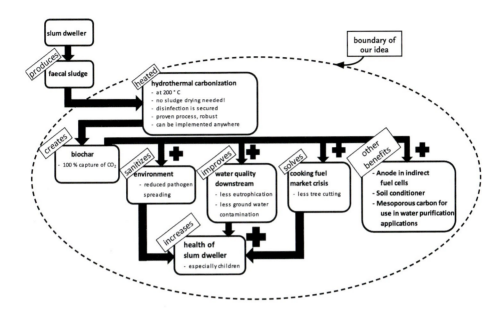

Figure 3. Improved sanitation in slums by using faecal sludge as a starting material for hydrothermal carbonisation, producing biochar that can create many beneficial impacts for the slum dwellers. Described further in detail in Katukiza et al. (2012).

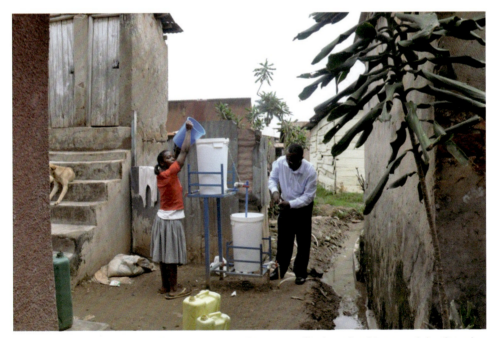

Figure 4. Improved sanitation in slums by using a two-step pilot grey water filter for nutrient (nitrogen and phosphorous) and pathogen removal, installed in Bwaise III slum (Kampala, Uganda). Described in detail in Katukiza et al. (2014a).

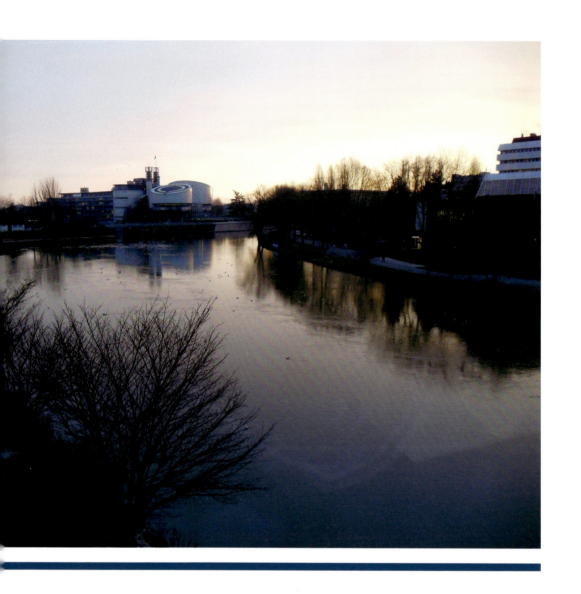

HYDROPOWER – SUSTAINABILITY, SECURITY OF SUPPLY, AND SYSTEM STABILITY

Achim Kaspar (COO VERBUND AG),
Andreas Kunsch (Advisor of the COO VERBUND AG)

Nowadays the whole global energy market is changing rapidly, however, electricity is already the backbone of our lives and is still becoming even more important from day to day. By today, everyone should be aware that energy from renewable sources will and has to be our future and that hydropower is the renewable world champion. Furthermore, it will be the catalyst of our energy transition.

General price levels – not only regarding fossil fuels – increased massively, thus, the pressure on our society as well as on the economy is increasing more and more, and because of the current negative impacts, the big question is when the necessary price level stabilisation will happen. In theory the transformation of our energy system to a more sustainable and ecological one has already been sketched; however, the present situation is becoming even more difficult, and the truth is, that under the current settings and changes we don't know any more for real, how long this transformation will in fact take.

As shown in the diagram below, the worldwide electricity generation in 2020 measured approx. 26.800 TWh, but only about 28 % of the amount was produced from regenerative resources.

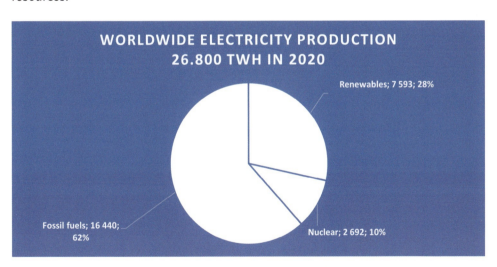

62% had fossil origins, accounting for 16.440 TWh, including coal (9.467 TWh), natural gas (6.257 TWh), and oil (716 TWh). Furthermore, 10% (2.692 TWh) was produced by nuclear power. However, nowadays renewable resources are becoming even more important than they have been before.

Of the approx. 28% made up of renewable electricity production worldwide (7.593 TWh), 16% was generated from hydropower, only 6% from wind power plants, and a further 3% from solar power plants, and 3% from bioenergy. (1)

Therefore, hydropower is the most important renewable technology for our worldwide low-carbon electricity generation. In detail, the major part – 58% – of the worldwide renewable electricity production was produced by hydropower, with an output of 4.347 TWh. Furthermore, 21% was generated by wind power plants (1.596 TWh), 11 % by solar power plants (833 TWh), and the remaining 10% by bioenergy (709 TWh) (1).

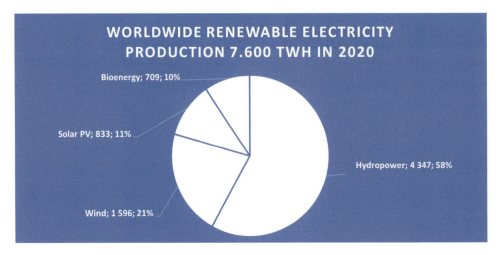

"During 2021 – 2030, annual gross hydropower generation is expected to increase by almost 850 TWh (+19%) globally, with China alone accounting for more than 42% of this growth and India, Indonesia, Pakistan, Vietnam and Brazil together contributing another 21%." (2)

Looking at the European Union, the electricity production in 2019 (2) was approx. 2.904 TWh, of this amount only approx. 35% of the electricity was generated regeneratively. However, about 38% of the entire amount of electricity (1.112 TWh) was produced by fossil fuels and approx. 26% by nuclear power (765 TWh). (3)

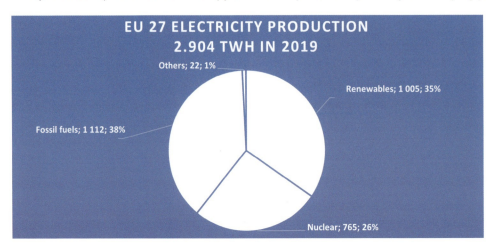

Of the entire amount of electricity produced (1.005 TWh) within the European Union, only 13% was produced from wind power, 12% from hydropower plants, 4% from solar power plants, 4% from bioenergy, and 2% from geothermal supplies. A major part of the renewable electricity generation within the European Union in 2019 (1.005 TWh) was produced from wind power (367 TWh, 42% of all renewables). A further 39% was generated from hydropower plants (345 TWh), 12% from solar power plants (125 TWh), and the remaining 6% from bioenergy (55 TWh). (4)

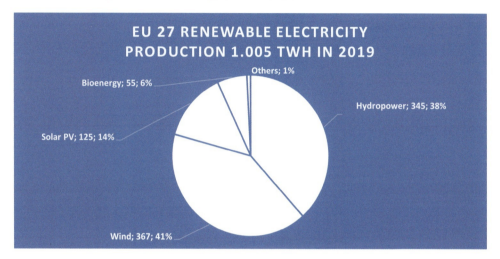

Furthermore, hydropower is not only the most mature and most popular technology for renewable electricity production worldwide, but its advantages, qualities, and power spectrum are manifold:

- Hydropower is a sustainable, local, and national form of production and has a noticeable global development potential;
- it is mandatory to reach the sustainable development goals for SDG 7 clean energy, SDG 12 responsible production, and SDG 13 climate action by compensating fossil fuels, but beyond this it also supports the other sustainable development goals;
- hydropower plants have the highest efficiency and a maximum of flexibility within the renewable family and are very important for true independence from fossil energy;
- there are 3 types with different advantages: run-of-river power plants can generate electricity through natural water flow; reservoir power plants are able to store electricity by keeping water for several days, months, or even years; pumped storage power plants can store electricity by pumping water from a lower reservoir to a higher reservoir at times when enough electricity is produced and therefore they can generate electricity at times of high demand or when supply from other plants is not possible;
- run-of-river, reservoir, and pumped storage plants together guarantee the security of the electrical supply by low-carbon electricity generation;

- it has a high rate of guaranteed capacity (in comparison to wind and solar power plants), depending on the type of hydropower plant, a secure performance from 45 to 90% can be expected, looking at the combined Austrian and German territory, this equals an output of about 70% (5). In contrast, other renewable energy sources have much lower secure performance values, eg. wind power or photovoltaic, as they depend on the availability of wind and sunshine.
- it is the most efficient large-scale technology to store electricity short-, medium- and long-term. Storage power plants will play an ever increasingly important role in our future energy systems as they are necessary to integrate the renewable energy from wind and solar power plants;
- hydropower is the only renewable technology supplying a significant performance as well as a huge number of system services for the net companies: backup of the primary electrical supply through providing the base load as well as the peak load feed-in; the possibility to compensate differences between schedules and forecasts; the compensation of power station failures; the possibility to compensate for varying demands and supplies of electricity, thus providing system stability; the ability for black-starts after a black-out, hence protecting the security of power supply;
- hydropower operators are partners in regions and respected employers and can play an important role for flood control;
- according to the net-zero emissions scenario from International Energy Agency, hydropower is the backbone of the global electricity security and the most cost-effective, dispatchable, and flexible low carbon electricity technology option to integrate variable renewable energy shares;
- beyond the production of electricity, water storage reservoirs are used worldwide for important tasks such as holding back precipitations and irrigations as well as being reservoirs for drinking water – one of the most fundamental elements of human life.

The global pandemic, interrupted supply chains, and current conflicts show us how sensitive our global markets are, especially the energy market. Hydropower is a reliable technology, which can help us to become a more sustainable world in the future. It´s clear that all power plant projects have to be developed under actual legal principles, but it´s also clear that there is no project or plant without at least a minimum impact on nature. Of course it is necessary to mitigate these impacts to have the best outcome for the energy supply and climate. However, we have to balance and compare the impacts on the local environment and the advantages for the climate in general, for all projects under discussion as well as existing power plants.

In the Hydropower Special Market Report, a publication from the International Energy Agency, seven policy recommendations are stated:

- "Move hydropower up the energy and climate policy agenda
  Sustainably developed hydropower plants need to be recognised as renewable energy sources. Governments should include large and small hydropower in their long-term deployment targets, energy plans, and renewable energy incentive schemes, on a par with variable renewables. ...
- Enforce robust sustainability standards for all hydropower development with streamlined rules and regulations
  Environmental and sustainability regulations for new and existing hydropower projects need to be streamlined to provide developers with clear rules and reasonable implementation timelines, without compromising stringency. ...
- Recognise the critical role of hydropower for electricity security and reflect its value through remuneration mechanisms
  Policy makers should assess and recognise the full electricity security and system stability value of hydropower and should translate these benefits into remuneration schemes that make new projects and modernisation activities bankable. ...
- Maximise the flexibility capabilities of existing hydropower plants through measures to incentivise their modernisation
  Governments should better recognise the value of dispatchable renewable energy and encourage modernisation and refurbishment investments, for instance through loan guarantees or by providing long-term revenue certainty. ...
- Support the expansion of pumped storage hydropower
  Governments should consider PSH plants as an integral part of their long-term strategic energy plans, aligned with wind and solar PV capacity expansion. Policy makers should identify suitable undeveloped sites and choose installations that would have the least environmental impact, for example closed-loop systems and the adding on of PSH capabilities to existing infrastructure such as abandoned mines, natural reservoirs and established reservoir plants. It is also essential to clarify the regulatory environment for storage by standardising definitions and eliminating double grid tariffs. ...
- Mobilise affordable financing for sustainable hydropower development in developing economies
  Governments, international financial institutions, and development agencies should support public-private partnerships and mobilise low-cost capital to de-risk hydropower projects in developing countries. ...
- Take steps to ensure to price in the value of the multiple public benefits provided by hydropower plants
  Governments should develop metrics to assess the multipurpose value of hydropower dams and recognise the net economic and social benefits of water management services to local communities. ..." (6)

As the consumption of electricity will grow rapidly, it is necessary that we optimise the existing hydropower plants and develop further available potentials as well as possible for a sustainable low carbon industry. To be able to reach this goal in the near and not in the distant future, experts, lawyers, and politicians are absolutely asked to evaluate, optimise, and adapt the huge number of different laws and rules as well as to assure a faster path for approvals. Otherwise, it will not be possible to reach our ambitious goals on time.

REFERENCES

(1) World Energy Outlook 2021, 2021, International Energy Agency, page 307, Web download 22.04.2022: https://iea.blob.core.windows.net/assets/4ed140c1-c3f3-4fd9-acae-789a4e14a23c/WorldEnergyOutlook2021.pdf

(2) Hydropower Outlook 2021, 2021, International Energy Agency, page 73, Web download 22.04.2022: https://iea.blob.core.windows.net/assets/4d2d4365-08c6-4171-9ea2-8549fabd1c8d/HydropowerSpecialMarketReport_corr.pdf

(3) EU energy in figures – Statistical Pocketbook 2021, 2021, Publications Office of the European Union, page 94,Web download 22.04.2022: https://op.europa.eu/en/publication-detail/-/publication/41488d59-2032-11ec-bd8e-01aa75ed71a1/language-en

(4) EU energy in figures – Statistical Pocketbook 2021, 2021, Publications Office of the European Union, page 95,Web download 22.04.2022: https://op.europa.eu/en/publication-detail/-/publication/41488d59-2032-11ec-bd8e-01aa75ed71a1/language-en

(5) Markus Pfleger, Hans-Peter Ernst, Klaus Engels, Rudolf Metzka, 2015, Guaranteed capacity of hydro power plants in Germany and Austria, VGB PowerTech Journal, 9/2015, page 30-33, VGB PowerTech Service GmbH, Deilbachtal 173, 45257 Essen, Germany, http://www.vgb.org

(6) Hydropower Outlook 2021, 2021, International Energy Agency, Chapter 5 – Policy Recommendations, page 113-118 , Web download 22.04.2022: https://iea.blob.core.windows.net/assets/4d2d4365-08c6-4171-9ea2-8549fabd1c8d/HydropowerSpecialMarketReport_corr.pdf

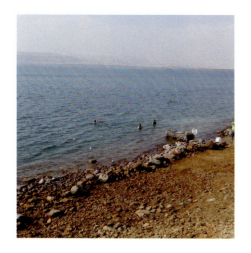
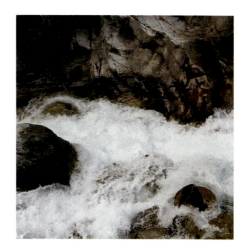
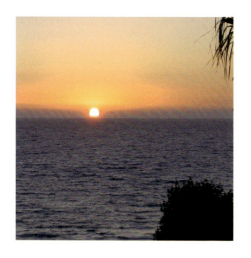
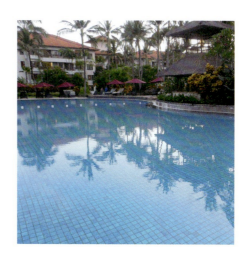
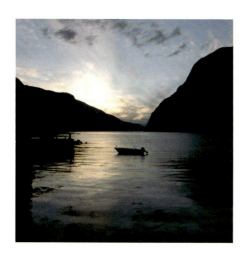
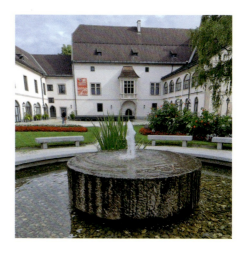

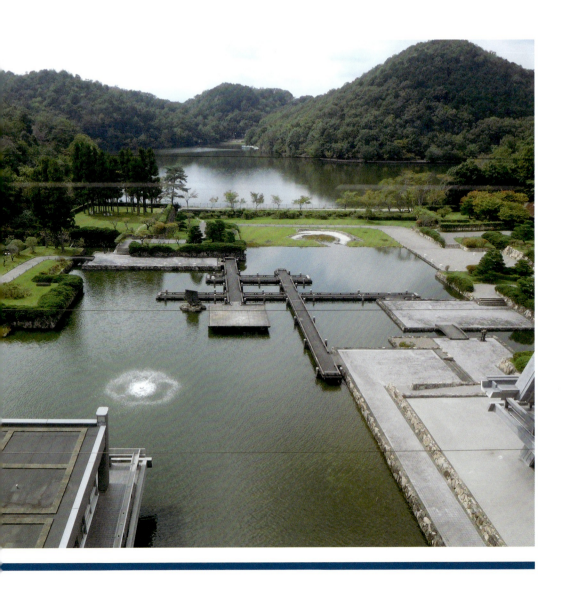

POTENTIALS FOR ENERGY-GAINING OUT OF WATER & WASTEWATER TREATMENT PLANTS

Josef Schnaitl (Gisaqua GmbH)

These days water and energy are turning out to definitely be the most critical resources on our blue planet. Due to growing population and industrial demands, water needs to be treated more and more to avoid or decrease pollution on the one hand and to provide the various water quality requests – most important for drinking water – on the other hand. As water treatment is consuming significant amounts of energy, it is obvious to seek and use opportunities to save or substitute this energy within the plant areas which are most effective, because beside saving energy, it reduces the infrastructural needs for energy supply and distribution.

Such opportunities have been given and have already been successfully implemented to some extend but not to the extent that it seems to be possible and necessary. The following categories seem to be worthwhile to be developed further:
- Use of biological energy contained in water
- Use of energy from level or pressure difference
- Additional use of used space

List of shortcuts used in the following:
- WWTP   wastewater treatment plant
- DWTP   drinking water treatment plant
- PE   people equivalent
- TPD   tons per day, plant capacity
- HEPP   hydroelectric power plant
- CoGen   combined generation unit (heat & electrical energy)
- PV   photovoltaic
- kWp   Kilo watt peak (max. module power)

USE OF BIOLOGICAL ENERGY CONTAINED IN WATER

This potential of energy is addressed for wastewater treatment plants. The necessary reduction of a potentially high content of carbon can be separated and transferred to digesters (liquid fermenters) where it is converted to biogas (methane). This process is well developed and has proven the effective and reliable operation from small size plants of 10.000 PE up to > 4 mio PE. Sources of carbon are:
- Fat and grease removed at inflow
- Sludge out of pretreatment, thickened up to 8%
- There is also the possibility to add shredded biologic waste and increase biogas production.

The gained biogas is stored in gas tanks and converted to electrical and heat energy in CoGen units as per the actual needs of the plant. The implementation provides the following positive effects:

- Heat energy is used to heat the sludge to and in the digester and excess-energy can be used for feeding district heating networks.
- The potential of electrical energy production is able to cover the demand of the plant up to and above 100 %.
  - The expectable power rating is around 300 kW per 100.000 PE

A quite large application of this kind of energy gaining was installed in the Vienna Main Treatment Plant >4 mio PE (finished in 2020) and is operating successfully. It is well documented on the homepage under www.ebswien.at/klaeranlage.

USE OF ENERGY OUT OF LEVEL OR PRESSURE DIFFERENCE

This potential of energy gaining can be implemented in numerous cases within the plant concept. One common application is the energy recovery in RO-plants which gains energy from pressure reduction from high pressure of up to 70 bar by pressure-exchanger or turbines or return-fed pumps. These applications are obligatory as they return >25% of the energy.

- The principal of gaining energy from pressure differences can also be applied in many other cases.

A rarely used opportunity of energy gaining is using level differences. Many water sources are based on dam reservoirs. This water most likely needs to be treated in DWTP´s and their possible location is normally at much lower levels compared to the dam level. A level-difference of 50 m (equal to 5 bar pressure) is quite normal.

As a DWTP needs a zero-pressure in the inflow, the pressure of say 5 bar needs to be reduced to zero. This energy potential can be gained in a HEPP by turbines.

To enable the adaption of the HEPP to the different dam levels (dry and wet season) and the different flows (high and low water consumption), return-fed pumps with variable speed drives are applied. A configuration could be (already installed):

- 3 pumps (return feed) with 1.1 Megawatt output
- 3 frequency converters 1.2 MW
- Level and flow control unit for the optimisation of treatment capacity and energy production
- Bypass configuration for emergency cases

This configuration is based on common market products which ensures sustainable operation and best available service and maintenance support.

The potential of a DWTP with a capacity of 300,000 TPD and a level difference of 50m on average reaches a capacity of around 3 Megawatt max., which can substitute the plant-energy-need to a certain extend.

ADDITIONAL USE OF USED SPACE

Beside the demand of energy water treatment plants require a relatively large area. This area can and should be also used for energy production out of photovoltaic. Typically, the following spaces are subject to use:

- Roofs of buildings
- Carports
- Treatment basins

Application on roofs and carports are common practice.

There are more and more upcoming intentions to cover treatment basins of WWTP´s to

- Reduce or avoid odour
- To avoid spreading viruses (a known an issue since Covid 19)

The sense of covering DWTP-basins could be to avoid the warming of water and to avoid algae growth

Given the facts, it seems to be logical to combine these intentions with the implementation of photovoltaic plants.

For example, the scale of basins at mid and larger sized WWTP´s is normally in the range of 60x10 meters. This area enables a PV capacity of around 60-80 kWP.

- A mid-size plant with 6 basins can provide 350-500 kWp.
- This represents a yearly production of 300,000 to 500,000 kWh.

With the optimised orientation of PV modules, the energy production in the summertime is quite harmonic to the energy needs of a WWTP. Even if the energy potential in the winter is quite low, there is a very valuable contribution to the energy demand of a plant.

As always, to use these opportunities, there are some challenges which have to be addressed and solved:

- Corrosive atmosphere has to be considered (Ammonia, H_2S, Chlorine)
  - There are smart solutions to address this issue
- Potential of ex-zones need to be considered
  - This needs to be addressed together with corrosive atmospheres

- Service access to the machinery in the basins has to be enabled, solved through
  - Defined service entrance areas
  - Mobile PV module design, modules can be withdrawn and basins are fully accessible

CONCLUSION

Beside optimised process solutions, the need for establishing smart and sustainable energy concepts is becoming obligatory for every new and existing treatment plant. In this regard it should be considered that there are also further opportunities to optimise the energy balance of water treatment plants This is an essential need to provide the next generations with the basic needs of life – **WATER and ENERGY.**

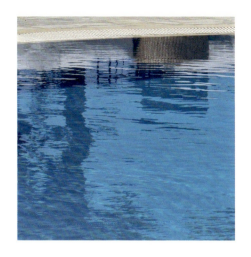
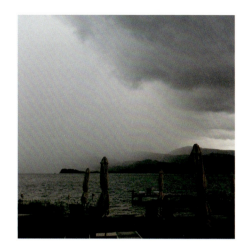
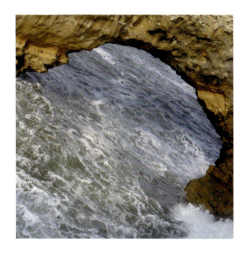
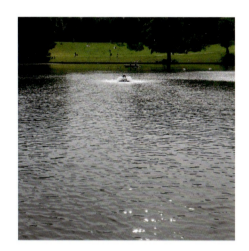
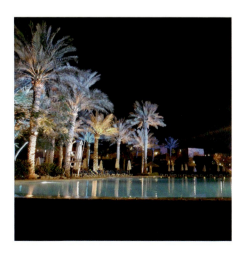
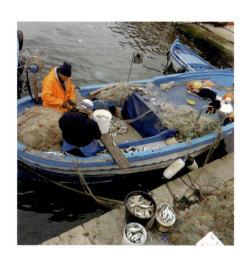

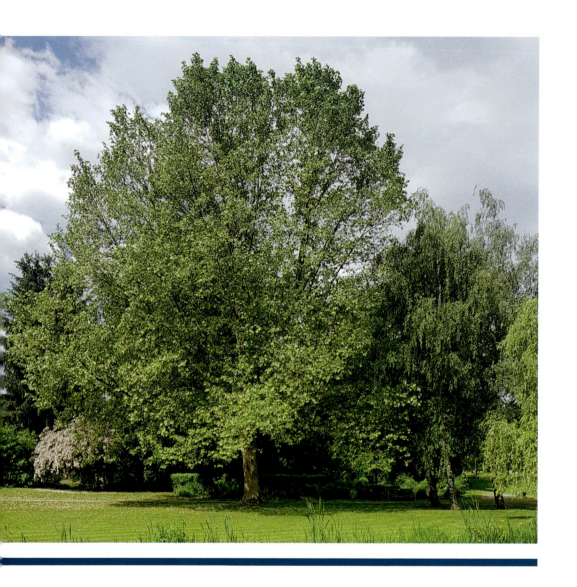

THE QUEST FOR A BIODIVERSE
WATER FUTURE IN EUROPE

Sara Eeman (Aveco de Bondt, The Netherlands), Mona Arnold (VTT Technical Research Centre of Finland),
Piia Leskinen (Turku University of Applied Sciences, Finland), Natasa Mori (National Institute of Biology, Slovenia),
Sanja Gottstein (University of Zagreb, Croatia), Sacha de Rijk (Deltares, The Netherlands)

EUROPEAN WATER HISTORY

Water quality and biodiversity have been a focus of attention in Europe for decades. The year 1970 marks the moment when the European Communities passed the first law to protect the environment. The principle of "the polluter pays" was introduced. At that time, there were only six Member States, so the measure had little effect on water quality across Europe. That has changed over the years with the steady expansion of this partnership to the now 27 Member States. The most important framework that has actively managed water quality across the EU since the year 2000 is the Water Framework Directive (WFD). This means that the principles and goals of European water quality management are regulated in detail and implemented in a controlled manner under the supervision of the Commission.

CONTEXT

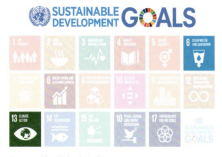

Source: The United Nations

The purpose of this chapter is to find answers to the challenges and outline solutions (tech and non-tech innovations) and best practices related to biodiversity recovery in (and near) water. The context encompasses the Water Framework Directive (Europe) as well as the UN directed SDGs 6 and 13: "Cleaner Water and Sanitation" and "Take urgent action to combat climate change and its impacts." Where Natura2000 areas overlap with water bodies, the context is broadened to more specific habitat goals, requiring a fit-for-purpose water quality and quantity.

WE VISION

In Europe, Water Europe is the voice and promoter of water-related innovation and RTD in Europe. The ambition is to shorten the path between the development of new methods and techniques and their introduction in the market for the benefit of better water quality. Water Europe has set out a blueprint for a society in which "the true value of water is recognised and realised, and all available water sources are managed in such a way that water scarcity and the pollution of water are avoided, water and resource loops are largely closed to foster a circular economy and optimal resource efficiency," while the water system is resilient against the impact of climate change events. Biodiversity is an important indicator for achieving these goals.

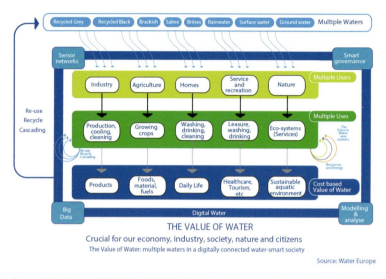

THE VALUE OF WATER

Crucial for our economy, industry, society, nature and citizens

The Value of Water: multiple waters in a digitally connected water-smart society

Source: Water Europe

Source: Water Europe, THE VALUE OF WATER: https://watereurope.eu/wp-content/uploads/2020/04/WE-Water-Vision-english_online.pdf.

THE ROLES OF BIODIVERSITY

Freshwater ecosystems host exceptional biodiversity: covering less than 1% of the Earth's surface, they conceal more than 10% of all species, including one-third of all vertebrate species (Strayer and Dudgeon 2010). A significant amount of these species remains unexplored so far (Cantonati et al., 2020). Despite their critical importance, the biodiversity crisis impacts freshwater ecosystems most significantly. From 1970 onwards, the surface of natural wetlands shrank by 35% (3 x the rate of forest loss), and a progress in sustainably managed water resources needs to double to achieve 2030 aims (2021 Report on SDG 6). Progress towards safeguarding key biodiversity areas has stalled over the last 5 years, only 42% of key global freshwater biodiversity areas has been protected (2021 Report on SDG 13). The direct, instantaneous effects of biodiversity decline on aquaculture and fishery are caused by both the quantity and quality deficiencies of fresh water. The former also effects agriculture where as this depends on irrigation. In the longer term (decades), both contamination and over-use of groundwater, leading to deeper groundwater levels endangers primary production as well as drinking water supply. Hydropower is an important clean source of energy, increasing in importance with the decreased use and availability of fossil fuels. However, in too many instances these infrastructures have a strong negative effect on the biodiversity, due to the obstacles in the water as well as not meeting minimal flow requirements (Gracey & Verones, 2016).

Biodiversity is a system-indicator, telling us about the actual suitability for aquatic life, water quality, and ecosystem health. Decrease in water-related biodiversity is a result of a combination of issues such as pollution, climate change, over-use, etc. The other way around, healthy, biodiverse freshwater ecosystems directly or indirectly support ecosystem services such as flood control, water retention, water purification, nutrient cycling, food supply (aquacultures, fisheries), etc.

FRAMEWORK FOR ACTION

The Water Framework Directive requires EU Member States to achieve good status in all bodies of surface water and groundwater by 2027. A good status refers to the ecological and chemical status of surface waters as well as the chemical and quantitative status of groundwater. From these components, the ecological quality of the surface water shows very limited improvements. The WFD is the largest coherent standard water programme in the world based on a legal framework to which EU member states have committed themselves. Although WFD was not designed specifically to increase biodiversity as such, it provides Europe with a strong weapon to take serious action on water related ecosystems and the accompanying biodiversity. Actions should therefore focus on this in particular in the coming years. To improve biodiversity, we need an integrated approach, in which measures should above all be systemic (e.g. on a catchment-scale).

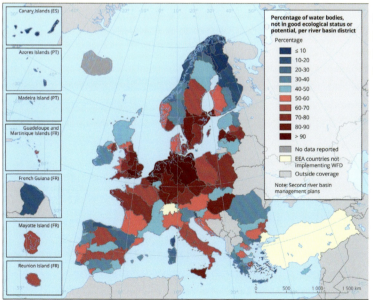

Source: European Environment Agency (EEA): https://www.eea.europa.eu.

AN EFFECTIVE APPROACH

We see important solutions in a more system-driven approach to the problem. We distinguish four different types of instruments

- **Instruments that support the analysis** of the problem and thereby provide insight into a possible action perspective to support the formulation of actions.
- **Tools that assist in sustainable solution design** at the level of sewerage systems, regional scales, and river basin level.
- **Modern digital knowledge management** tools (such as Digital Models, Digital Shadows, or Digital Twins) that help underpin effective decisions and actions.
- **Innovative partnerships** such as Water-oriented Living Labs (WoLLs), whereby biodiversity objectives can be pursued effectively and transparently for stakeholders in a Nexus context.

ACTION READINESS

For each of these instrument types, a lot are already available. Speeding up their use and implementation is needed to start making a difference. Examples of existing technology which can be upscaled are: remote sensing measurement techniques that provide information about the chemical/physical status of water that influences biodiversity or e-DNA monitoring techniques that provide rapid, reliable information on the species in a waterbody. For digital knowledge management, several platforms are forming and have been formed that link data and enable the step from data to information and required action on a large scale, in a dynamic environment (e.g. BIOMONDO).
Since all this is already available, let's:

- Take advantage of having the outlines of an emergency plan available, e.g. An Emergency Recovery Plan for Freshwater Biodiversity.
- Identify on which terrains technical tools are insufficient in order to focus research in those directions. We think here of the quantification of populations in an automatic way and the short comings of large scale monitoring, which is needed to get a firmer grip on the development of larger areas.
- Propose involvement of leaders and engineers responsible for implementation at all levels. WOLL's are a very useful instrument in this, which can be applied both EU-wide and city-wide, increasing the awareness needed to make the shift towards sustainability in the broad (Nexus) sense. Of course, many trainings, games, etc., exist as well: creating overviews, of what to apply where and on which level, can speed up their implementation.

We can start applying the available tools and fit gaps and new questions requiring research within actual projects. These projects/Living Labs are aimed to improve water-related biodiversity, allowing learning on the job and involving all stakeholders, as was done within, for example the **Marker Wadden project**. This will increase biodiversity as well as awareness and provide developers and researchers with the information and support to fill in the missing knowledge and tools. These can eventually be used to further speed up towards biodiversity, indicating a resilient water system everywhere.

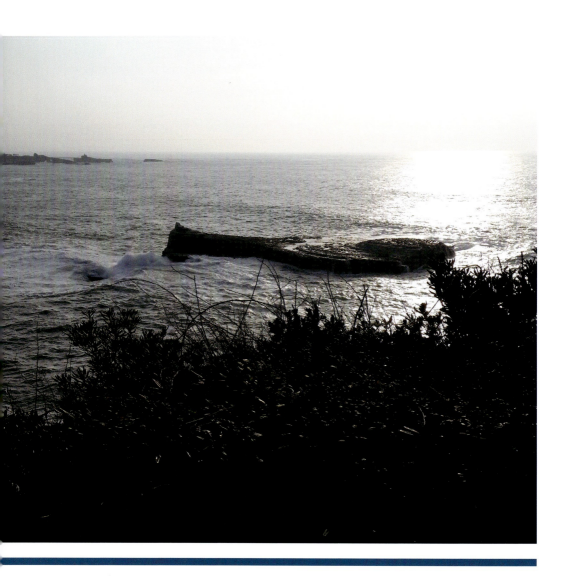

GLOBAL WATER SECURITY CHALLENGES AND SOLUTIONS

Dragan Savic (KWR Water Research Institute, The Netherlands; Centre for Water Systems, University of Exeter, United Kingdom),
Milou M.L. Dingemans (KWR Water Research Institute, The Netherlands; Institute for Risk Assessment Sciences, Utrecht
University, The Netherlands), Ruud P. Bartholomeus (KWR Water Research Institute, The Netherlands; Soil Physics and Land
Management, Wageningen University & Research, The Netherlands)

INTRODUCTION

Global water security is a multi-dimensional and enduring human goal. These multiple dimensions reflect human aspiration to manage risks related to water, including droughts, floods, landslides, desertification, pollution, epidemics, and diseases, as well as disputes and conflicts. As our water resources are becoming more scarce and polluted, ensuring sufficient clean water is a major global challenge, in line with the sustainable development goal (SDG) for clean water and sanitation (SDG 6). It can be argued that water plays a role in all 17 SDGs, but particularly for the following goals it is clear that they will not be met if sufficient clean water is not available: SGD1 (No Poverty), SDG2 (Zero Hunger), SDG3 (Good Health and Well-being), SDG8 (Decent Work and Economic Growth), SDG11 (Sustainable Cities and Communities), SDG13 (Climate Action), SDG14 (Life Below Water), and SDG15 (Life on Land). Major transitions are needed to enable the protection and sustainable management of our water resources. This requires research, innovation, valorisation, governance, and the development of knowledge and skills in the global water sector.

This chapter presents three interrelated global water security challenges and potential solutions that can contribute to achieving water-related SDGs, and in particular the SDG6.

WATER AVAILABILITY AND REUSE

Population growth and economical growth result in increasing water resource demands. Additionally, climate change increases the uncertainty about the availability of conventional water resources like groundwater, surface water, and precipitation (Pronk et al., 2021; Wada & Bierkens, 2014). In many regions, groundwater overexploitation is a major risk for future water availability (de Graaf et al., 2019; Wada & Bierkens, 2014). Even in areas with a yearly precipitation surplus, we are increasingly confronted with drought damage in agriculture and nature as well as increasing pressure on the availability of water for high-grade applications such as the production of drinking water (Brakkee et al., 2022; Klijn et al., 2012; Pronk et al., 2021). In temperate climates, groundwater resources will generally not be depleted. However, only a small part of the total groundwater stored can be exploited sustainably, i.e. without causing damage to other functions, like nature.

Even flood-prone areas like those in the Netherlands, which for many decades focused on discharging water in order to prevent waterlogging and flooding (de Wit et al., 2022), were facing serious drought damage in the years 2018-2020 (Brakkee et al., 2022; Philip et al., 2020; van den Eertwegh et al., 2021). For Europe, the drought of 2018-2020 has been identified as the new benchmark for what we may expect for the future climate (Rakovec et al., 2022). Therefore, strategies are being developed to control the risks of water shortages and to secure long-term supplies of clean freshwater for all sectors. Such strategies include increasing regional self-sufficiency in meeting the demand for fresh water and improving the utilisation of the available water sources, including those that are currently non-conventional. Together with the current drive towards a circular economy (Morseletto et al., 2022), this urges the continued exploration of the potential for and applicability of (treated) effluent as an alternative water source, i.e. wastewater reuse.

Although the natural water system and municipal water cycle / water chain are traditionally considered separate systems, they are strongly physically connected: the natural water system forms the resource for anthropogenic use, while waste products of anthropogenic origin are emitted from the water cycle into the water system. Opportunities for increased water availability can however be found when the natural water system is considered, together with the municipal water cycle, as a truly integrated system (Pronk et al., 2021). Cross-sectoral approaches in which the water chain and water system are truly integrated are gaining attention, as cross-sectoral water reuse has the potential to substantially reduce the demand for groundwater and surface water (Figure 1, Pronk et al., 2021). However, risks and trade-offs throughout the whole water system need to be identified: practical and governmental challenges arise when innovations are integrated in the context of regional water systems. Therefore, the potential of water reuse schemes, e.g. for irrigation and water suppletion, needs to be evaluated in a global, national and regional context, to i) identify how reused water propagates through the water system and ii) quantify the reduced pressure on water resources. Besides water-quantity based analysis, water quality demands, health and safety aspects, technological requirements, regulations and public perception need to be considered (Dingemans et al., 2020). An integrative context is thus essential for the responsible implementation of water reuse for a robust water supply.

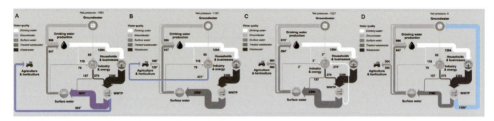

Figure 1: Potential of cross-sectoral water reuse to reduce the use of groundwater resources (figure adapted from Pronk et al., 2021; http://creativecommons.org/licenses/by/4.0/).

WATER QUALITY CHALLENGES, INCLUDING PMT (PERSISTENT, MOBILE, AND TOXIC) SUBSTANCES

Besides having an impact on water availability, population growth, a growing economy, and climate change also have a major impact on the quality of water bodies and drinking water sources (Ryberg and Chanat 2022; Sjerps et al., 2017; Wolf and van Vliet 2021). Nutrients (phosphorus and nitrogen) and anthropogenic chemicals continue to be emitted into the aquatic environment, and climate changes may result in favourable growing conditions for (opportunistic) pathogens (Nijhawan and Howard, 2022). As the number of chemicals that are used and produced worldwide increases and chemicals are constantly being replaced by others, the number of chemicals that can end up in the environment, including the water system, keeps increasing.

The Water Framework Directive and Drinking Water Directive have set clear goals and targets, and many different stakeholders and authorities with different responsibilities are needed and have to work together to achieve better environmental water quality. This requires practical and policy measures to protect and improve environmental water quality. In the Netherlands, several initiatives have followed from the Delta Approach to Water Quality (Delta Aanpak Waterkwaliteit, 2016), such as the national working group on Emerging Substances (Aanpak Opkomende Stoffen) and the aim to ban harmful chemicals (Substances of Very High Concern) from the environment by reducing the release of such chemicals from industrial activities. Recently, a science-to-action research programme was initiated by water authorities and drinking water companies and has developed user-friendly tools founded on existing scientific knowledge to support decision-making on measures to improve water quality (www.kiwk.nl). These types of activities in policy and practice need to be expanded across all EU Member States. As water pollutants are easily moving over national borders, transnational collaboration is particularly necessary for surface water quality protection. This has already led to the development of the NORMAN network, a network of universities and research institutes that collaborate and inform policy-makers on environmental monitoring including EU water quality (Dulio et al., 2020).

Drinking water companies guarantee that amounts of substances and microorganisms meet the requirements for safe and healthy drinking water. As the water system can be impacted by many different emissions, the drinking water sector puts a lot of effort into understanding the quality of its sources (RIWA-Meuse, 2022; Sjerps et al., 2019; Hartmann et al., 2021). Academic and applied research in collaborative research programmes inform water utilities on the quality of sources and the efficacy of management measures if problematic substances are detected. This is a good foundation for addressing water quality hazards, exposure patterns, and potential risks – also in the context of the use of alternative water sources and water reuse (Dingemans et al., 2020). Analytical methods that are developed in the context of risk-based monitoring (RBM) of water quality can support the assessment of environmental or health risks associated with water reuse and using alternative water sources by revealing their specific contamination patterns. Target chemical analyses that provide quantitative levels of chemicals that can be compared to safe levels are complemented with screening approaches to detect unknown and new chemicals of emerging concern (CECs); non-targeted chemical analyses (Béen et al., 2021), and effect-based monitoring of low-level mixtures (EBM) (Dingemans et al., 2019; Robitaille et al., 2022). With increased pressure on freshwater sources that are used for many different applications, it can be helpful to develop specific fit-for-purpose water quality standards for low- to high-grade applications.

Drinking water companies have developed monitoring and treatment strategies to deal with changes in water quality in their sources. A particular and current challenge that needs to be addressed, also in an integrated evaluation of water reuse and the use of alternative water sources, is the occurrence of persistent and mobile substances that are retained in and may propagate in the water system (Hale et al., 2022; Sims et al., 2022; Vughs et al., 2019). With the ambition to reduce the adverse environmental impact of persistent bioaccumulative chemicals, a process was set in motion to produce more mobile substances for many types of use. This has resulted in a substantial load of the water system with persistent and mobile substances, including per- and polyfluoroalkyl substances (PFAS). Many efforts are ongoing in EU member states and the water sector to deal with the large-scale pollution and remediation of the water system from these types of substances, and a general EU ban has been proposed. For this particular, very large group of PMT substances, it is recognised that a group-wise approach for monitoring and regulation is appropriate, as it is not feasible to address each of them one by one (Cousins et al., 2020). As such, a sum parameter for PFAS has been proposed for inclusion in the Water Framework Directive, and PFAS are included as two group parameters in the revised Drinking Water Directive, 'PFAS Total' and 'Sum of PFAS' (EC, 2020a). Before these parameters can be applied, technical guidelines regarding methods of analysis for monitoring still need to be established by the European Commission in the coming years. In the Netherlands, a REP approach has been proposed, in analogy to the Equivalency Approach for dioxins, for the risk assessment of all PFAS via all exposure sources (Bil et al., 2021). Research efforts are targeted toward analytical methods, improving the maturity of the REP values for PFAS and relative contributions of different exposure routes.

Group-wise regulation is also in line with the increased consideration of the fact that humans and the environment are exposed to complex low-level mixtures, consisting of different substances and changing over time. Although risk assessment and risk characterisation are traditionally applied substance-by-substance, European authorities aim to improve the risk assessment and sustainability of chemicals for authorisation by considering aggregate and mixture exposures, in line with the EU Chemicals Strategy for Sustainability (EC, 2020b).

To safeguard the environment as well as the production of safe and healthy drinking water and to support decision-making in complex societal and legislative challenges such as those related to water scarcity, circular economy, and the energy transition, it is critical to know which chemicals are present in the water system and if their levels can be expected to contribute to exposure and adverse effects on human health or the environment. Going into a future that will confront us with many water challenges and a continuing need to monitor and interpret water quality issues when addressing these challenges, it is critical to develop a European framework that considers current and future exposure patterns from different sources and the potential risks of low-level mixtures (Vermeulen et al., 2020) to decide on priorities in risk management and mitigation to protect human health and the environment.

DIGITAL WATER TRANSFORMATION OF WATER SERVICES

The last few decades have seen an unprecedented impact of modern digital technologies and the "digital transformation" of almost every element of our society (e.g. banking, transportation, tourism, and entertainment). While digital banking, transport apps (e.g. Uber), tourism platforms (e.g. AirBnB, Booking.com), and video and music streaming services (e.g. Netflix, Spotify), have disrupted traditional sectors, improvement of the planning and management of global water-related risks through digital transformation has been slow (Savic, 2022). The amount of information available today is unprecedented in human history, with 90% of it having been created only in the last two years. There is almost nothing we cannot measure, sense, or monitor, including many aspects relevant to water availability and water quality. The question is, how is the digital transformation of the water sector going?

The digital transformation in the water sector has been largely influenced by the scientific field of "hydroinformatics" (Savic, 2022). In the past, hydroinformatics was often referred to as a technology that applied ICT and artificial intelligence (AI) to complex water and societal challenges, but it is much more than that. Hydroinformatics can be considered a management philosophy, which is designed to tackle global water challenges and is enabled by technology (Savic, 2022).

The concept of hydroinformatics has its origins in computational hydraulics (Abbot, 1991) and dates back to times even before digital computers, e.g. electric-analogue groundwater models of the late fifties and early sixties. Since the proliferation of desktop computers in the early eighties, hydroinformatics tools and methods have increasingly found their application in the water sector leading to modern digital technologies being actively used for supporting planning and management decisions. The following outlines some of those technologies and applications.

AI and Machine Learning (Savic, 2022) applications have improved leakage management (i.e. detection and localisation) in water distribution systems. This is done by predicting future demand values and comparing them with the actual consumption to indicate a potential leak (Romano et al., 2010). Nature-inspired computing (e.g. genetic algorithms, particle swarm optimisation) is another AI methodology that has received a lot of attention and provides solutions for the planning and management of complex water systems (Maier et al., 2014).

A **Digital Twin** (Savic, 2022) is a replica of a physical system in a digital form. The key origins of the digital twin approach are in modelling and simulation (Conejos Fuertes et al., 2020). What is new about the digital twin is the real-time (and/or near real-time) information that is used to update it. This makes a digital twin a true reflection of the dynamics of the physical system. This type of modelling has the potential to change the decision support and management of water systems from reactive to proactive.

Augmented, mixed, and/or virtual reality technologies, collectively known as **Extended Reality** (Savic, 2022), can provide the augmented view of buried water infrastructure and locate possible problems and solutions or can be used to provide training for personnel in a safe (virtual) environment. Utility personnel can better engage in this safe virtual environment that protects them from the risk of injury or endangerment. Remote site data visualisation and ease of access to quality control information at remote sites through extended reality means also that operating costs can be reduced.

Serious games have recently made progress in tackling problems in environmental and water management fields (Savic, 2022). Their applications draw inspiration from training games, such as flight simulators or education and consensus-building games (Savic et al., 2016). While entertainment is not the main purpose of serious games, they allow players to experience interactively and visually some of the challenges facing water managers and policymakers in tackling droughts, flooding, or implementing water reuse and recycling.

Digital portals and online dashboards can help in engaging water users and empower them towards more sustainable behaviour (Savic, 2022). This approach is important not only to change attitudes toward resource wastage and demand management (Savic et al., 2014) but also to prolong the life of expensive infrastructure. Performance monitoring and data visualisation in a control room of a water utility could be also enhanced by AI/Machine Learning technologies by providing predictive analytics (Savic, 2022).

Remote sensing (Savic, 2022) by ground-based, airborne, and space-based sensors and platforms can provide a large amount of data for water resource management. Agricultural applications are the obvious example where monitoring water use efficiency is essential (Blatchford et al., 2019). The overuse of water in agriculture is of particular interest because about 70% of the world's freshwater withdrawals are for agriculture.

While *robotics* has found applications in manufacturing, healthcare, and disaster management, it has not penetrated the field of water management. Efforts are, however, underway to bring advanced robot technologies to water infrastructure management (Savic, 2022). The idea of a robot that is equipped with various sensors to collect data from an infrastructure system is not new. However, Van Thienen et al. (2018) have gone further by envisaging a robot that, once inserted into the pipe system, can remain permanently in it, can be recharged remotely, and can keep sending information about the condition of the system without the need for it to be taken out.

CONCLUSIONS

Future water management challenges related to climate change, including water reuse for a robust freshwater supply, and pollution of freshwater sources, are increasingly complex and interdependent, which makes it nearly impossible to make informed decisions without using digital tools. However, using these tools in isolation, i.e. without: i) using a proper conceptualisation of the water system as a whole, ii) taking advantage of various data streams and expert knowledge, will not lead to disruptive innovation breakthroughs in water management. Informed decisions need to be made also with respect to the protection of the environment from pollution and safeguarding the production of safe and healthy drinking water in a changing world that confronts us with complex societal and legislative challenges such as those related to water scarcity, circular economy and the energy transition. Hydroinformatics, as a management philosophy, is the key enabler for integrating data across data silos and providing data analytics that improves knowledge and eventually leads to making informed decisions.

REFERENCES

Abbot, M.B., 1991. Hydroinformatics. Information Technology and the Aquatic Environment, Avebury Technical, pp.1-85628.

Been F, Kruve A, Vughs D, Meekel N, Reus A, Zwartsen A, Wessel A, Fischer A, Ter Laak T, Brunner AM. Risk-based prioritization of suspects detected in riverine water using complementary chromatographic techniques. Water Res. 2021 Oct 1;204:117612. doi: 10.1016/j.watres.2021.117612.

Bil W, Zeilmaker M, Fragki S, Lijzen J, Verbruggen E, Bokkers B. Risk Assessment of Per- and Polyfluoroalkyl Substance Mixtures: A Relative Potency Factor Approach. Environ Toxicol Chem. 2021 Mar;40(3):859-870. doi:10.1002/etc.4835.

Blatchford, M.L., Mannaerts, C.M., Zeng, Y., Nouri, H. and Karimi, P., 2019. Status of accuracy in remotely sensed and in-situ agricultural water productivity estimates: A review. Remote sensing of environment, 234, p.111413.

Brakkee, E., van Huijgevoort, M.H.J., Bartholomeus, R.P., 2022. Improved understanding of regional groundwater drought development through time series modelling: the 2018–2019 drought in the Netherlands. Hydrol. Earth Syst. Sci., 26(3): 551-569. DOI:10.5194/hess-26-551-2022

Conejos Fuertes, P., Martínez Alzamora, F., Hervás Carot, M. and Alonso Campos, J.C., 2020. Building and exploiting a Digital Twin for the management of drinking water distribution networks. Urban Water Journal, 17(8), pp.704-713.

Cousins IT, DeWitt JC, Glüge J, Goldenman G, Herzke D, Lohmann R, Miller M, Ng CA, Scheringer M, Vierke L, Wang Z. Strategies for grouping per- and polyfluoroalkyl substances (PFAS) to protect human and environmental health. Environ Sci Process Impacts. 2020 Jul 1;22(7):1444-1460. doi: 10.1039/d0em00147c.

de Graaf, I.E.M., Gleeson, T., van Beek, L.P.H., Sutanudjaja, E.H., Bierkens, M.F.P., 2019. Environmental flow limits to global groundwater pumping. Nature, 574(7776): 90-94. DOI:10.1038/s41586-019-1594-4

de Wit, J.A., Ritsema, C.J., van Dam, J.C., van den Eertwegh, G.A.P.H., Bartholomeus, R.P., 2022. Development of subsurface drainage systems: Discharge – retention – recharge. Agric Water Manag, 269: 107677. DOI:https://doi.org/10.1016/j.agwat.2022.107677

Delta Aanpak Waterkwaliteit 2016. Intentieverklaring Delta-aanpak Waterkwaliteit en Zoetwater tussen overheden, maatschappelijke organisaties en kennisinstituten (Declaration of intent Delta Approach to Water Quality and Freshwater between governments, civil society organisations and knowledge institutes).

Dingemans MM, Baken KA, van der Oost R, Schriks M, van Wezel AP. Risk-based approach in the revised European Union drinking water legislation: Opportunities for bioanalytical tools. Integr Environ Assess Manag. 2019 Jan;15(1):126-134. doi: 10.1002/ieam.4096.

Dingemans MML, Smeets PWMH, Medema G, Frijns J, Raat KJ, van Wezel AP, Bartholomeus RP. Responsible Water Reuse Needs an Interdisciplinary Approach to Balance Risks and Benefits. Water. 2020; 12(5):1264. https://doi.org/10.3390/w12051264.

Dulio, V., Koschorreck, J., van Bavel, B. et al. The NORMAN Association and the European Partnership for Chemicals Risk Assessment (PARC): let's cooperate!. Environ Sci Eur 32, 100 (2020). https://doi.org/10.1186/s12302-020-00375-w.

EC (European Commission). 2020a. Directive (EU) 2020/2184 of the European Parliament and of the Council of 16 December 2020 on the quality of water intended for human consumption. https://eur-lex.europa.eu/eli/dir/2020/2184/oj.

EC (European Commission). 2020b. Chemicals strategy – The EU's chemicals strategy for sustainability towards a toxic-free environment https://environment.ec.europa.eu/strategy/chemicals-strategy_en.

Hale, S.E., Neumann, M., Schliebner, I. et al. Getting in control of persistent, mobile and toxic (PMT) and very persistent and very mobile (vPvM) substances to protect water resources: strategies from diverse perspectives. Environ Sci Eur 34, 22 (2022). https://doi.org/10.1186/s12302-022-00604-4.

Hartmann J, Chacon-Hurtado JC, Verbruggen E, Schijven J, Rorije E, Wuijts S, de Roda Husman AM, van der Hoek JP, Scholten L. Model development for evidence-based prioritisation of policy action on emerging chemical and microbial drinking water risks. J Environ Manage. 2021 Oct 1;295:112902. doi: 10.1016/j.jenvman.2021.112902.

H.R. Maier, Z. Kapelan, J. Kasprzyk, J. Kollat, L.S. Matott, M.C. Cunha, G.C. Dandy, M.S. Gibbs, E. Keedwell, A. Marchi, A. Ostfeld, D. Savic, D.P. Solomatine, J.A. Vrugt, A.C. Zecchin, B.S. Minsker, E.J. Barbour, G. Kuczera, F. Pasha, A. Castelletti, M. Giuliani, P.M. Reed, 2014. Evolutionary algorithms and other metaheuristics in water resources: Current status, research challenges and future directions. Environmental Modelling & Software, 62, pp.271-299.

Klijn, F., van Velzen, E., ter Maat, J., Hunink, J., Baarse, G., Beumer, V., Boderie, P., Buma, J., Delsman, J., Hoogewoud, J., 2012. Zoetwatervoorziening in Nederland: aangescherpte landelijke knelpuntenanalyse 21e eeuw, Deltares.

Morseletto, P., Mooren, C.E., Munaretto, S., 2022. Circular Economy of Water: Definition, Strategies and Challenges. Circular Economy and Sustainability: 1-15.

Nijhawan A, Howard G. 2022. Associations between climate variables and water quality in low- and middle-income countries: A scoping review. Water Research 210:117996.

Philip, S.Y., Kew, S.F., van der Wiel, K., Wanders, N., van Oldenborgh, G.J., 2020. Regional differentiation in climate change induced drought trends in the Netherlands. Environmental Research Letters, 15(9): 094081.

Pronk, G., Stofberg, S., Van Dooren, T., Dingemans, M., Frijns, J., Koeman-Stein, N., Smeets, P., Bartholomeus, R., 2021. Increasing Water System Robustness in the Netherlands: Potential of Cross-Sectoral Water Reuse. Water Resources Management: 1-15.

Rakovec, O., Samaniego, L., Hari, V., Markonis, Y., Moravec, V., Thober, S., Hanel, M., Kumar, R., 2022. The 2018–2020 Multi-Year Drought Sets a New Benchmark in Europe. Earth's Future, 10(3): e2021EF002394.

Romano, M., Kapelan, Z. and Savić, D.A., 2010. Real-time leak detection in water distribution systems. In Water Distribution Systems Analysis 2010 (pp. 1074-1082).

RIWA-Meuse. 2022. Drinking water relevant substances in the Meuse 2021. RIWA-Maas (RIWA-Meuse).

Vereniging van Rivierwaterbedrijven (Association of river water companies) (2016).

Robitaille J, Denslow ND, Escher BI, Kurita-Oyamada HG, Marlatt V, Martyniuk CJ, Navarro-Martín L, Prosser R, Sanderson T, Yargeau V, Langlois VS. Towards regulation of Endocrine Disrupting chemicals (EDCs) in water resources using bioassays – A guide to developing a testing strategy. Environ Res. 2022 Apr 1;205:112483. doi: 10.1016/j.envres.2021.112483.

Ryberg KR, Chanat JG. Climate extremes as drivers of surface-water-quality trends in the United States. Sci Total Environ. 2022 Feb 25;809:152165. doi:10.1016/j. scitotenv.2021.152165.

Savic, D., Vamvakeridou-Lyroudia, L. and Kapelan, Z., 2014. Smart meters, smart water, smart societies: The iWIDGET project. Procedia Engineering, 89, pp. 1105-1112.

Savic, D.A., Morley, M.S. and Khoury, M., 2016. Serious gaming for water systems planning and management. Water, 8(10), p. 456.

Savic, D., 2022. Hydroinformatics: Solutions for global water challenges. Hydrolink 2, pp. 48-49.

Sims JL, Stroski KM, Kim S, Killeen G, Ehalt R, Simcik MF, Brooks BW. Global occurrence and probabilistic environmental health hazard assessment of per- and polyfluoroalkyl substances (PFASs) in groundwater and surface waters. Sci Total Environ. 2022 Apr 10;816:151535. doi: 10.1016/j.scitotenv.2021.151535.

Sjerps RMA, Kooij PJF, van Loon A, Van Wezel AP. Occurrence of pesticides in Dutch drinking water sources. Chemosphere. 2019 Nov;235:510-518. doi:10.1016/j. chemosphere.2019.06.207.

Sjerps RMA, Ter Laak TL, Zwolsman GJJG. Projected impact of climate change and chemical emissions on the water quality of the European rivers Rhine and Meuse: A drinking water perspective. Sci Total Environ. 2017 Dec 1;601-602:1682-1694. doi: 10.1016/j.scitotenv.2017.05.250.

Van Thienen, P., Bergmans, B. and Diemel, R., 2018, July. Advances in development and testing of a system of autonomous inspection robots for drinking water distribution systems. In WDSA/CCWI Joint Conference Proceedings (Vol. 1).

Bil W, Zeilmaker M, Fragki S, Lijzen J, Verbruggen E, Bokkers B. Risk Assessment of Per- and Polyfluoroalkyl Substance Mixtures: A Relative Potency Factor Approach. Environ Toxicol Chem. 2021 Mar;40(3):859-870. doi:10.1002/etc.4835.

van den Eertwegh, G., de Louw, P., Witte, J.-P., van Huijgevoort, M., Bartholomeus, R., van Deijl, D., van Dam, J., Hunnink, J., America, I., Pouwels, J., 2021. Droogte in zandgebieden van Zuid-, Midden-en Oost-Nederland: het verhaal-analyse van droogte 2018 en 2019 en bevindingen: eindrapport, KnowH2O.

Vermeulen R, Schymanski EL, Barabási AL, Miller GW. The exposome and health: Where chemistry meets biology. Science. 2020 Jan 24;367(6476):392-396. doi:10.1126/science.aay3164.

Vughs D, Baken KA, Dingemans MML, de Voogt P. The determination of two emerging perfluoroalkyl substances and related halogenated sulfonic acids and their significance for the drinking water supply chain. Environ Sci Process Impacts. 2019 Nov 1;21(11):1899-1907. doi: 10.1039/c9em00393b.

Wada, Y., Bierkens, M.F.P., 2014. Sustainability of global water use: past reconstruction and future projections. Environmental Research Letters, 9(10): 104003. DOI:10.1088/1748-9326/9/10/104003.

Wolff E, van Vliet MTH. Impact of the 2018 drought on pharmaceutical concentrations and general water quality of the Rhine and Meuse rivers. SciTotal Environ. 2021 Jul 15;778:146182. doi: 10.1016/j.scitotenv.2021.146182.

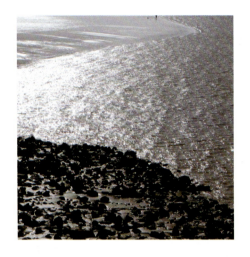
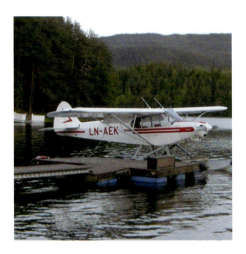
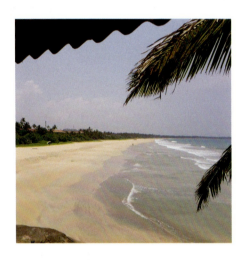
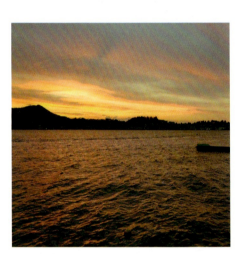
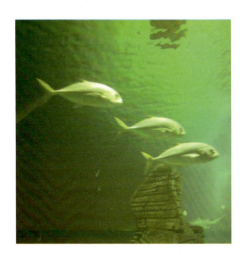
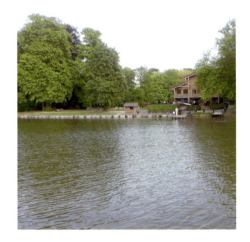

TECHNOLOGY, ENGINEERING AND EDUCATION

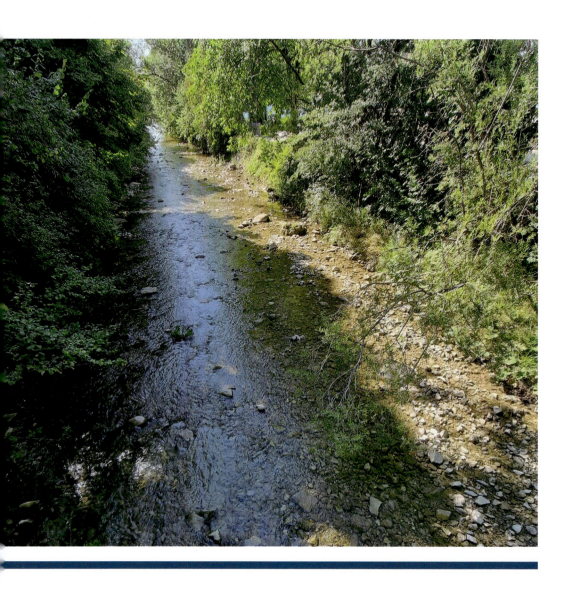

WATER-ORIENTED LIVING LABS

Andrea Rubini (Director of Operations at Water Europe)

WHAT IS A WATER-ORIENTED LIVING LAB?

A Living Lab is not only a network of infrastructures and services, but also a collaborative ecosystem that is established to sustain community-driven innovations in a multi-stakeholder context. It offers an effective research methodology for sensing, prototyping, validating, and refining innovative solutions in multiple and evolving real-life contexts. The Living Lab concept is hence highly relevant to the innovation process leading towards a **Water-Smart Society**. A (Water-Oriented) Living Lab takes research and development out of laboratories and sets it in real-life contexts. This allows for a better understanding of what triggers innovation and helps identify those innovations that prove to be successful in different environmental, social, and cultural – collaborative and inclusive – water contexts towards the achievement of the goals represented in the SDG6 and SDG17.

The European history of Living Labs traces its roots to the Scandinavian cooperative and participatory design movement of the 60s-70s, the European social experiments with IT in the 80s, and the Digital City projects of the 90s. During the 90s, the digital city concept took hold in Europe and elsewhere, referring to several digital initiatives undertaken by cities, especially related to digital representations of the city, digitally related economic development and urban regeneration initiatives, and the provision of internet access for citizens. By the early 2000s, consistent European Union (EU) policies lead to the Finnish presidency launching the European Network of Living Labs (ENoLL) on the 20th of November 2006.

Since then, Living Lab initiatives and communities have had a significant impact on European research and innovation policy, migrating from more linear research and innovation approaches to open and collaborative innovation concepts. Not only did these developments influence the research agendas and programmes of the European Union (e.g. EU R&D Framework programmes, Horizon 2020 and currently Horizon Europe), they also inspired research, development, and innovation at the regional level within Cohesion Policy and Territorial Cooperation Programmes, particularly through the Smart Specialisation Strategies defined for all EU Regions and Member States.

Living Lab initiatives in Europe often start from the needs and aspirations of local and regional stakeholders. They provide valuable input to European policies and programmes, including Horizon 2020 and Horizon Europe, Smart Specialisation, the Urban Agenda, Cohesion Policy, and so forth.

Specific calls for proposals in different sections of the European Research and Innovation programmes directly recommend Living Labs as innovation and experimentation instruments in areas related to smart cities, urban innovation, mobility, and international cooperation. Living Labs are promoted to combine vertical domains of research (health, smart cities, climate, water, education, etc.) with horizontal and territorial aspects (digitalisation, multi-stakeholder governance, etc.) to strengthen the emerging European Open Innovation ecosystem. The aim is that Living Labs enable the more effective resolution of societal challenges, acceleration of innovation, internationalisation of industries (e.g. SMEs), and the creation of a pan-European experimentation environment supporting the realisation of the European (Digital) Single Market.

WATER EUROPE PROGRAMME FOR WATER ORIENTED LIVING LABS

In 2018 Water Europe launched the initiative to **map and promote a network of Water-Oriented Living Labs** (WOLLs) as a means for sharing and collaborating to foster common methodologies and tools across Europe that support, stimulate, and accelerate co-creative innovation processes, relying on users' involvement with the final aim to tackle urgent societal challenges resulting amongst others from climate change and to contribute to future EU Policies such as the Green Deal through a Water-Smart Society. In 2019 the **Atlas of EU Water-Oriented Living Labs** was published. The Atlas counted more than 100 WOLLs with different levels of operational capacity and maturity.

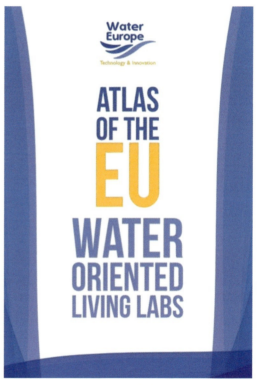

This initiative aimed at representing a means for sharing and fostering common methodologies and tools across Europe that support, stimulate, and accelerate co-creative innovation processes, relying on users' involvement with the final aim to tackle urgent societal challenges resulting amongst others from climate change and to contribute to EU Policies and transformation such as the joint Green and Digital transitions through a Water-Smart Society.

Taking a closer look at the characteristics of WOLLs as described above, six aspects (or foundational elements) represent the essential characterisation of a Living Labs: user involvement, service creation, infrastructure, governance, innovation outcomes, methods, & tools.

Hence, we can characterise a Water-Oriented Living Lab more in detail as follows:

- **USER INVOLVEMENT**
  Objective: involve users of water (e.g. urban/citizens, industry, and/or agriculture) as well as users of innovations that enable a "Water-Smart Society" (e.g. same as above + utilities and related service providers such as waste water management companies, etc.), giving them the opportunity to influence the solution that will affect their life later on.

- **SERVICE CREATION**
  Objective: facilitating and supporting the development of new ideas, services, and solutions that contribute to a sustainable and Water-Smart Society and offering representative (semi) real-life environments of water production, distribution, and (re) use, for co-design and validation.

- **INFRASTRUCTURE**
  Objective: providing the physical or virtual environment, to integrate, try-out, validate, and measure the performance of water innovations. This may include an experimental set-up (e.g. in labs or demo-sites) or (preferably) real-life test environments including (external) infrastructures for water production, distribution, and (re)use (e.g. at utilities, urban areas, (agro) industrial sites).

- **GOVERNANCE**
  Objective: engage the quadruple helix from the water sector in a (inter) regional context e.g. involving public (water managing) authorities (including utilities), water users (e.g. cities/citizens, industries, and/or agriculture), water research organisations, and technology developers, which jointly agree on managing and maintaining the WOLL.

- **INNOVATION OUTCOME**
  Objective: facilitate predominantly innovations that contribute to a sustainable and Water-Smart Society ("mission focus"). These outcomes can be knowledge, new products and services, and/or IPR. Outcomes can be in the form of finished end-user applications but also in the form of prototypes or mere knowledge about usage patterns.

- **METHODS AND TOOLS**
  Objective: provide and continuously update specific (interoperable) methods and tools to acquire relevant large scale user data related to the targeted innovation outcomes within the water sector.

WATER EUROPE DEFINITION OF WATER-ORIENTED LIVING LABS

It is hence relevant to define the concept of a Water-Oriented Living Lab. Considering the specific features and characteristics of the water sector, as well as the goal to foster the longer-term vision of a Water-Smart Society, Water-Oriented Living Labs have been defined by Water Europe as follows:

Water-Oriented, real-life demonstration, and implementation instrument that brings together public and private institutions, government, civil society, and academia to 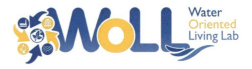 *jointly build structured grounds to develop, validate, and scale-up innovations that embrace new technologies, governance, business models, and advancing innovative policies to achieve a Water-Smart Society.*

As such WOLLs can be characterised by the type of collaborations and type of stakeholders involved, e.g. public–private–people partnerships quadruple/quintuple helix, as a model of open innovation and as eco-systems that foster cross-sectoral collaboration.

WHAT IS NEXT FOR WOLLS?

Water Europe has planned and organised resources to further develop and deploy the Water-Oriented Living Lab instrument in close collaboration with the EU co-funded partnership Water4All in the drive towards a Water-Smart Society.

The **Water4All Partnership**, cofunded by the European Union within the frame of the **Horizon Europe programme**, aims at enabling water security for all in the long 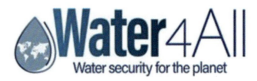 term through boosting systemic transformations and changes across the entire research – water innovation pipeline, fostering the matchmaking between problem owners and solution providers.

Water4All brings together a wide and cohesive group of **78 partners** from **31 countries** in the European Union and beyond. This consortium gathers a variety of partners from the whole water Research, Development and Innovation (RDI) chain.

Water Europe leads the Pillar D of Water4All which intends to demonstrate and scale up water innovations through the support of the existing Water-Oriented Living Labs, establishing new potential WOLLs in potentials territories and connect them in a collaborative Network of WOLLs to enhance long term sustainability and effectiveness.

To pursue WOLLs strategy in Water4All and as comprehensive action wider initiative, Water Europe updated the assessment methodology WOLLs from the ones used for the ATLAS published in 2019 and adopted the **Harmonization Cube**, tailored for the water sector with the future goal of a network of collaborative Water-Oriented Living Labs. To this end, Water Europe published two publications in 2022 that aim to define the practices and assessments methods of Water-Oriented Living Labs and provide a manual with a clear vision on how to assess and evolve WOLLs:

- Water-Oriented Living Labs: Notebook Series #1. Definitions, practices and assessment methods
- Water-Oriented Living Labs: Notebook Series #2. How to assess and evolve Water-Oriented Living Labs. A manual with a vision

Both publications will address the immediate challenge to stimulate and guide the growth and development of WOLLs along concrete steps towards a role in tackling all the challenges of the vision of a Water-Smart Society and towards a well-functioning WOLL with the highest level of maturity, a Water Europe LL (WELL).
This effort starts with the actions planned in the Pillar D of the partnership with Water4All.

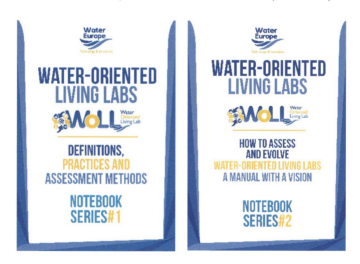

The ultimate objective for Water Europe is to develop a collaborative network of WELLs – or 'WELLNet' – which will make an indispensable contribution to realising Water Europe's Vision of a Water- Smart Society and contribute to the achievement of the SDG6 and SDG17.

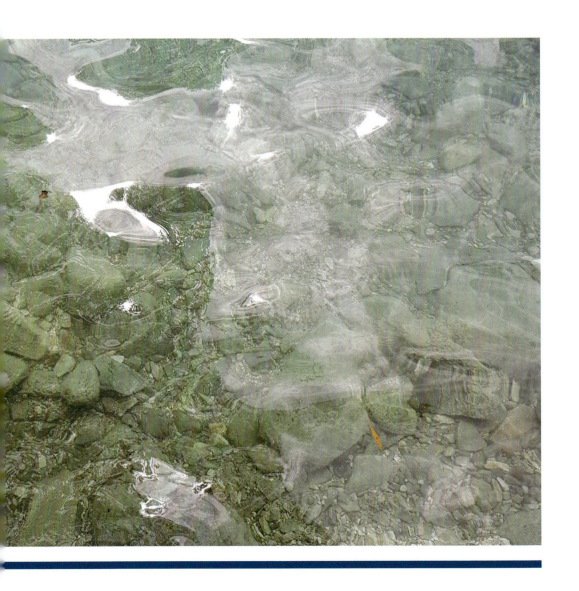

PROCESS SIMULATION – DIGITAL TWINS OF WATER TREATMENT PLANTS

Paul Schausberger (Managing Director UNIHA Wasser Technologie GmbH),
Peter Latzelsperger (Managing Director UNIHA Wasser Technologie GmbH)

INTRODUCTION

Pure water does not naturally exist on this planet, as all water resources are mixtures of water with other substances. The mixtures range from almost pure water in rain or ice caps to water containing high loads of salts, biogenic, and industrial matter. Clean and pure water; however, is not only vital as a primary source of life but has an impact on nearly every sustainability goal and development target of a society.

Traditionally, different approaches and parameters are used to characterise the composition of water mixtures in the potable, sewage, or industrial sectors. However, due to the pollution of the natural sources as well as the increasing demand for water reuse, a common language and denomination must be found. This common language supports the characterisation and comparison of different water types and its use/reuse across the industries.

"Process simulation is a model-based representation of chemical, physical, biological, and other technical processes and unit operations in software. Basic prerequisites for the model are chemical and physical properties of pure components and mixtures, of reactions, and of mathematical models which, in combination, allow the calculation of process properties by the software" (Wikipedia contributors, 2021).

In plant design, process simulation is used to model the treatment process and to calculate the relevant mass end energy balances. Based on these balances, the process can be evaluated in terms of the energy and chemical consumption as well as the by-product and waste flows. Those balances also form the basis of the treatment plant's Total Cost of Ownership (TCO) and the plant's ecological footprint.

Lately, such model-based representation is also referred to as a digital twin (Wikipedia contributors, 2022), which can contribute to the entire lifecycle of a treatment plant.

Considering the fact that wastewater treatment plants alone consume between 1-3% of the total energy consumption globally, the consideration of the lifecycle impact of plants is of key essence (Circular Economy: Tapping the Power of Wastewater, n.d.).

In general – in light of recent energy price increases as well as the necessity to reduce the energy consumption in terms of externally supplied energy (vs. energy recovery and sustainable energy components in situ), these concepts have increased in importance.

However, whereas commercial software tools are available for process simulation in selected industries. e.g. the petrochemical or power industry or municipal wastewater treatment, there is still demand for such tools for water engineering in general. Here, one main bottleneck is the missing universal model for the composition of water mixtures, as mentioned above.

DEVELOPMENT OF A NEW PROCESS SIMULATION TOOL

UNIHA provides water treatment solutions for all sectors and industries. Our mission is to provide our customers with solutions that are optimised for their individual case. Process simulation enables us to create those solutions and, together with the simulation specialists from SIMTECH (https://www.simtechnology.com/cms/), we have developed a relevant software tool.

In the first step, we have defined a model for the composition of water mixtures. Water mixtures are composed of pure water (H_2O) and non-water matter. This matter can comprise of almost all of the chemical elements as well as inorganic and organic molecules and aggregates:
- Inorganic ions, e.g. Na, Cl, HCO3, CO3, Ca, Mg...
- Inorganic gases, e.g. O2, CO2, NH3, H2S...
- Inorganic solids, e.g. CaCO3, SiO2, metal hydroxides...
- Organic molecules, e.g. methane, phenol, cyanide, pesticides, hormones...
- Organic macromolecules, e.g. carbohydrates, nucleic acids, proteins, lipids, mineral oil...
- Microorganisms, e.g. virus, bacteria, phytoplankton...
- Aggregates/Macroparticles: seaweed, plastic, hair...

It is impractical to balance all of the distinct elements for a treatment process, hence sum parameters are being used. We propose to define the composition by chemistry (inorganic/organic) and physical appearance (dissolved/suspended). This leads to the following composition matrix for the non-water matter (all variables in mg/kg of water):

	inorganic	organic	total
dissolved	IM_d	OM_d	W_d
suspended	IM_s	OM_s	W_s

In the second step, we have developed a model for the mixture mass density (ρ, kg/ m³) and heat capacity (c_p, J/kg/K) as a function of the composition model above. Both properties are required to describe the mass and energy balances.

Furthermore, we have investigated how to correlate the composition model with commonly used parameters such as Total Dissolved Solids (TDS), Dissolved Inorganic Carbon (DIC), Dissolved/Total Organic Carbon (DOC/TOC), Chemical Oxygen Demand (COD) and the elemental composition of Carbon-Nitrogen-Oxygen. These correlations allow for the input of field data from water analysis to the process simulation.

The third step was the modelling of the unit operations, i.e. the single treatment steps used for water treatment. For the first software version, we implemented the mass and energy balances for the following unit operations:
- Sedimentation
- Flotation
- Chemical and biological reactors
- Membrane and bed filtration
- Adsorption and ion exchange
- Reverse osmosis
- Sludge thickening and dewatering
- Heating/cooling
- Tanks, pumps, mixer/splitter

The resulting tool allows for the prediction of the mass and energy balances for every type of water treatment process; hence it forms the process digital twin:
First, the process is built graphically by arranging icons resembling the unit operations and connecting them by lines resembling the streams of matter. Next, the user needs to enter the basic settings such as composition, pressure, and temperature of the incoming streams or performance parameters for the unit operations. In the last step, the underlying equation system is solved and the simulation results are displayed.

In the following, we present selected UNIHA cases where the tool was used to identify the optimum treatment scheme and to provide the required data to design the plant equipment:

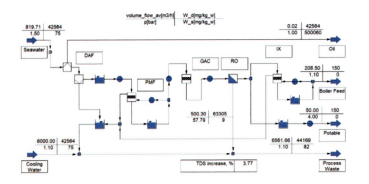

Figure 1: conversion of seawater to boiler feed and potable water; unit operations: dissolved air flotation (DAF), pressure media filter (PMF) with backwash, granular activated carbon filter (GAC), reverse osmosis (RO), ion exchange (IX), buffer tanks, pumping

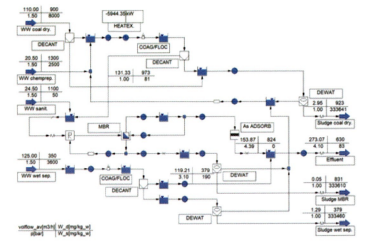

Figure 2: conversion of coal processing waste water for reuse or river discharge; unit operations: cooling (HEATEX), coagulation/flocculation (COAG/FLOC), sedimentation (DECANT), membrane bioreactor (MBR) with backwash, arsenic adsorber (As ADSORB), sludge dewatering (DEWAT), buffer tanks, pumping

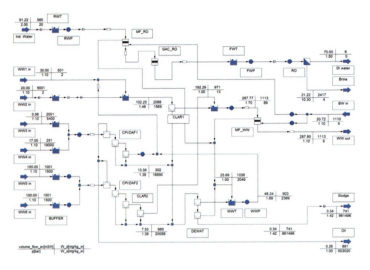

Figure 3: conversion of steel mill waste water for river discharge and conversion of river water to cooling system makeup; unit operations: oil separation (CPI), dissolved air flotation (DAF), pressure media filter (MF) with backwash, granular activated carbon filter (GAC), reverse osmosis (RO), sedimentation (CLAR), dewatering (DEWAT), buffer tanks, pumping

CONCLUSION AND OUTLOOK

The process simulation tool we have developed allows us to create better solutions for our clients and to move and act quicker. This gives us a clear competitive advantage and serves as a unique selling point. On a meta-level, our simulation tool also allows for a better understanding of mass-energy balances and, hence, quickly gives a base information which can serve to develop energy efficiency strategies, touchpoints for circular economy approaches, and holistic concepts for water resource management.

In light of a growing demand for clean water as well as possible add-on-usages for by-products from water treatment, such holistic concepts also gain more and more importance in an economic and business sphere. These add-on and re-use scenarios, e.g. brine mining for lithium, could yield business models which not only consider water treatment as such but also alternative options for the exploitation of by-products and, hence, a better Total Cost of Ownership balance of the total water treatment facility.

The future might also see a commercially available version of the simulation tool as well as the further integration of the process digital twins in the control and operation of UNIHA plants, e.g. the validation of field data with process simulation results.

SOURCES

Circular Economy: Tapping the Power of Wastewater. (n.d.). International Water Association. Retrieved 28 October, 2022, from https://iwa-network.org/learn/circular-economy-tapping-the-power-of-wastewater/

Wikipedia contributors. (2021, 24 April). *Process simulation.* Wikipedia. https://en.wikipedia.org/wiki/Process_simulation

Wikipedia contributors. (2022, 17 October). Digital twin. Wikipedia. https://en.wikipedia.org/w/index.php?title=Digital_twin

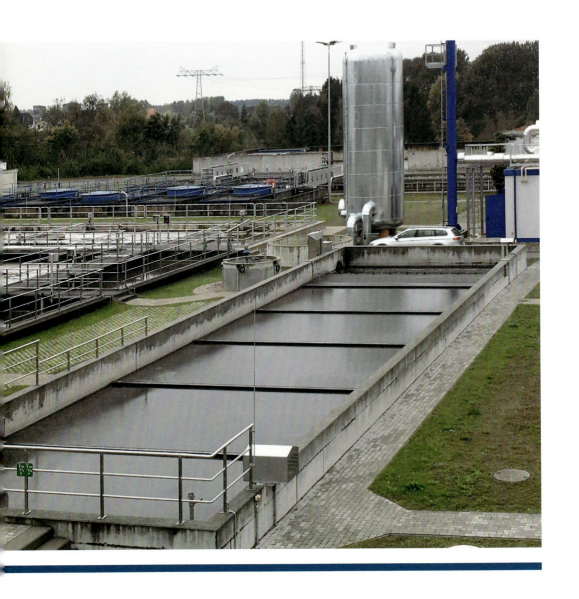

INNOVATIVE ENVIRONMENTAL
TECHNOLOGY MADE IN EUROPE

Augustin Perner (CEO at PROBIG GmbH)

**"Safe drinking water is cheap and obvious in Austria.
We're working hard to enable drinking water production and
an optimised water treatment all over the world."**

PROBIG® has been developing, planning, and producing high-quality chain scrapers, DAF, and API separators made of high-tech plastics for decades. As a pioneer of this technology, the company, which operates globally, is an international market leader and one of the most innovative suppliers of plastic chain scrapers for water and waste water technology.

The modern clarification and scraping systems combine the highest standards of environmental protection and certified quality with the best operational safety, as well as optimum cost and energy efficiency. With PROBIG®'s sustainable solutions, leading industrial companies and municipalities in more than 80 countries make an important contribution to reducing water consumption and ensuring an optimal water supply.

SUSTAINABLE ACTION AT ALL LEVELS

The issue of the environment is very important to PROBIG®. The company is clearly committed to the UN Sustainable Development Goals, and as a "Member of SDG 6," PROBIG® is fully committed to ensuring access to clean water and sanitation for all.
The company sets up activities along the entire value chain that help to protect the environment and resources and to make products and services holistically more sustainable, including:

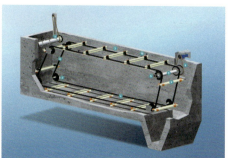

- Focus on state-of-the-art plastics technology,
- Energy-efficient component production,
- Selection of shipping companies based on reduced CO_2 emissions,
- Short shipping distances through regional (sub)suppliers,
- Upgrading the company fleet with electric vehicles,
- Energy generation at the Vöcklamarkt site with photovoltaics, and much more

Figure above: Belt scrapers made of high-tech plastics: innovative technology for the future
Figure on the left side: Wastewater treatment plant with chain

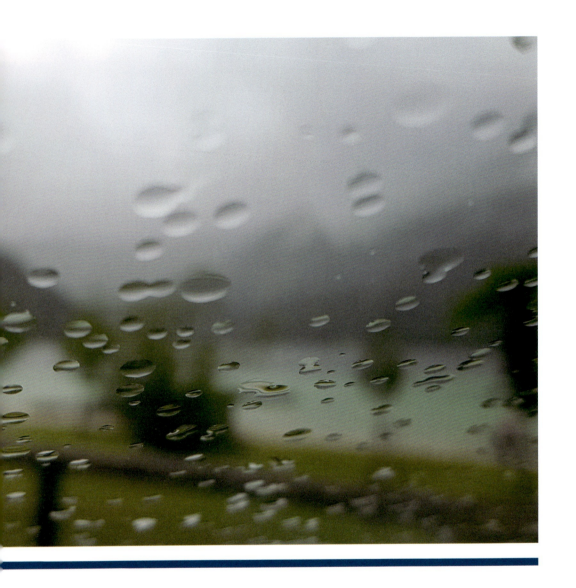

THE ROLE OF ADVANCED OXIDATION FOR THE PRODUCTION OF RE-USE WATER

Konrad Falko Wutscher
(Managing Director at SFC Umwelttechnik GmbH)

BACKGROUND

While a vast portion of mankind is still not being served by wastewater collection and treatment, wastewater treatment plants (acr. WWTPs) in developed countries observe the problem of lack of availability of sufficiently treated effluents apted for re-use as drinking water resources, as re-use water for technical and agricultural purposes, and as reclamation water for groundwater resources. Even the highly rated so-called tertiary treatment fearing nutrient removal is regarded as non-sufficient for higher level use purposes as indicated, not to speak of the long-term contamination potential of such treated effluents when applied to soils and water bodies.

These issues are well known, but strategies have hardly been focusing on the implementation of the so – called "quaternary treatment" (except in individual hot spots or in selected countries, e.g. Switzerland). The pollutants to be eliminated refer mainly to "pharmaceuticals and personal care products (acr. PPCPs).

However, such terms are unprecise and a bit euphemistic. Scientific literature refers to micropollutants, which appears to be a broader term rather than PPCP in view of the huge variety of compounds.

For example, about 4,000 different pharmaceutical ingredients are used in the EU, not including hundreds of different biocides, herbicides, pesticides, etc., which at an increased level find access and entry to the sewerage system. As a matter of fact, many of these compounds (some of these pre-degraded and transformed in the human body) pass into WWTPs which are unfit to degrade these typically refractory compounds and hence leave the plants more or less unchanged and / or not decreased to a decently low level.

Consequently, the micropollutants end up and accumulate in water and soil bodies showing various (long-term) effects which are only partly known and understood.

There is no doubt that in view of the increasing scarcity of unpolluted water, the issue of micropollutants and its elimination have a growing and decisive importance. Challenges are being described multifold by the enormous financial demands for removal, proving of technical viability, and finally the assessment of the long-term effects of the quaternary treatment of wastewaters on the environment.

STATE OF THE ART

The quaternary treatment of treated effluents in order to remove micropollutants (which typically are soluble rather than particulate – apart from very fine suspended solids or microplastics) mainly focusses on the combination of advanced oxidation by chemical oxidation agents followed by an adsorption stage (typically by AC activated carbon of many different styles, types, and selectivities).

The adsorption stage has turned out to be imperative as a kind of policing stage as the nature and actual composition of the transformation products (compounds) resulting from oxidation can be predicted neither in quantity nor in quality.

Such an adsorption stage will hence mitigate the eventual (long-term) negative effects of the very transformation products eventually arising in the finally treated effluents which leave the plants to the recipients or re-users. Nevertheless, the key process component is the AO advanced oxidation treatment stage.

Apart from generic AO applying classical chemical oxidation agents like H_2O_2, $KMnO_4$, or something similar (which have turned out to be by far too expensive and/or a secondary polluter), the AO technology used as a standard is ozonisation.

Ozonisation is effective but involves a number of disadvantages such as the necessary drying of atmospheric air before ozone generation, capsulation of the ozonisation facility and destruction of residual ozone, high power consumption, and rigorous safety regulations – not to speak of the high TOTEX of such facility.

A recently developed alternative to ozonisation is the production of ionised air as a non – thermal plasma out of non – pretreated atmospheric air.

INNOVATIVE IONISED AIR OXIDATION TECHNOLOGY

Similar to the production of ozone, ionised air is produced in a reactor featuring a high voltage corona discharge (DBD dielectric barrier discharge) employing a catalyst. Apart from the different isomeres of oxygen, which are produced in the presence of OH, radicals are the key factor for explaining the extra high oxidation potential over that of ozone.

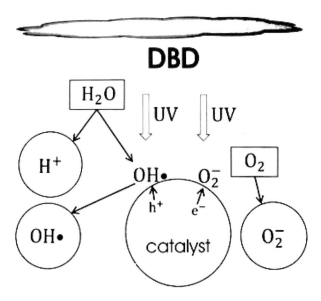

The main differences over ozonisation refer to different voltage levels, frequency, retention time, humidity, but especially to the presence of a catalyst.

The non – thermal plasma of ionised air needs to be applied as quickly as possible on the micropollutants given the very short lifetime of the OH radicals. This can be realised by a high-speed turbine which injects the plasma into the liquid media in a sufficiently rapid way.

The system of oxidation by ionised air is significally cheaper than an ozonisation plant both in terms of investment and especially of operation costs (here: of power costs which attain only around 60% of those of ozonisation).

A number of semi – technical and full scale applications have been launched and studied. These include the removal of micropollants (of selected pharmaceuticals such as Carbamazepin, Sulfomethaxol, and others), the destruction of microorganisms (which has the simultaneous effect of disinfection), and the oxidation of hardly oxidable elements like arsenic, manganese, and others).

With growing investments due to the need for high quality re-use water produced from treated effluents, a wider use of non – thermal plasma of ionised air can be expected.

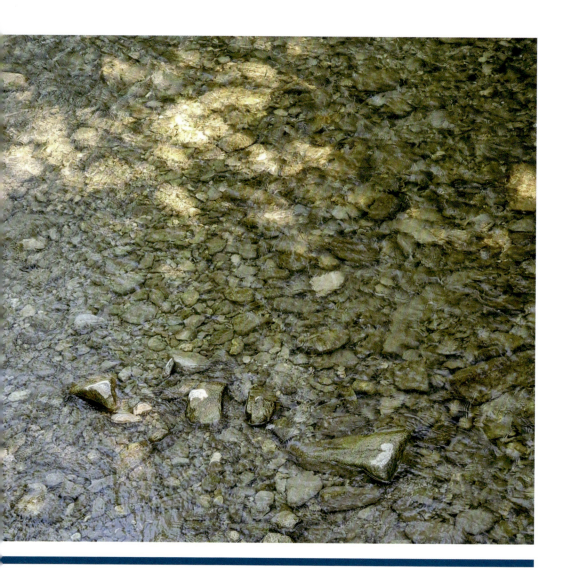

COLD PLASMA TO BATTLE PERSISTENT WATER POLLUTANTS

Juergen F. Kolb (Professor at INP Greifswald),
Klaus-Dieter Weltmann (Chairman of the Board and
Scientific Director at INP Greifswald)

EXECUTIVE SUMMARY

Water supply and wastewater treatment are at a very high level and quality in Europe. There are some new technological developments based on cold plasma treatment that are ready to enter the market and which could lead to an even higher quality of water supply and wastewater treatment.

The aim of this article is to draw attention to such new developments of water and wastewater treatment using various cold plasma applications and to encourage the discussion about setting up new or improved standards regarding the minimum requirements of water and wastewater treatment devices and even bigger production facilities.

This development is also supported by the increased availability of renewable energy sources such as wind and sunlight. Besides the need for effective and reliable devices, new methods and synergies between well-known and new technologies open up treatment possibilities with much higher cleaning results than before.

PERSISTENT AND EMERGING THREATS TO WATER RESERVOIRS

Despite the good standing and high quality of water supply and wastewater treatment in Europe, water resources and supplies are continuously being challenged by sustained and emerging threats. On the one hand, these are a consequence of advanced societies themselves, and, on the other hand, they have arisen from recent global developments, such as extreme weather events. Since the first alarming reports that even small concentrations of psychiatric drugs or oestrogens can have a significant environmental impact, e.g. on the behaviour and gender distribution of fish populations (Brodin et al., 2013; Purdom et al., 1994), pharmaceutical residues in particular have gained increasing scientific and public attention. Many of these compounds are rather stable and withstand conventional water treatment (Stackelberg et al., 2004; Ternes et al., 2002). In response to the potential risk, the European Commission added drugs that were already found in relative abundance in European surface waters – but especially diclofenac, 17α-ethinylestradiol, and 17β-estradiol – to a watchlist of emerging pollutants (European Parliament and Council of the European Union, 2013). After going into force, wastewater treatment plants were required to take measures to reduce the release of these substances. Another class of anthropogenic pollutants of growing concern is agrochemicals, particularly pesticides, which are still essential for successful farming in the industrialised and land-locked countries of the European Union. However, their burden on the environment and hazards for consumers have become evident (Devi et al., 2022; Kim et al., 2017). Therefore, the European Green Deal includes a substantial reduction in the future use of agrochemicals and especially pesticides (European Commission, 2022). Even when successfully implemented, different agrochemicals will remain for years to come, especially in soil from where they will percolate into groundwater or run off into surface water. The remediation of these substances faces the same issues that are experienced for pharmaceuticals. A popular example is the herbicide glyphosate (Jönsson et al., 2013). In addition to these man-made problems, natural toxins have recently been recognised as potential threats for the aquatic environment and the production of potable water (Hansen et al., 2021). Among this vast group of pollutants, cyanobacterial toxins have started to spoil surface waters even more frequently than before. This is caused by higher seasonal temperatures and the increasing eutrophication of water bodies, which promotes the proliferation of cyanobacteria. Although the microorganisms themselves are effectively removed by conventional water treatments, their toxins might persist. Accordingly, more advanced treatment options need to be deployed (Schneider & Bláha, 2020). The list of examples for the contamination of water resources can be easily expanded with other problematic substances, which have faded in and out of public attention over recent years. In part, this is due to advances in analytical methods, which revealed the occurrence of more and more compounds of concern at smaller and smaller concentrations. Concurrently, the monitoring of water resources, drinking water, and wastewater plant effluents has continuously expanded and several studies have provided comprehensive overviews for specific ecosystems, regions and countries (de Souza et al., 2020; Monteiro & Boxall, 2010). However, most of these pollutants are a result of the economics of thriving industrialised communities. This is, for instance, the case for the production, use, and disposal of synthetics, e.g. the release of plasticisers (bisphenols) or perfluorinated carbons (PFCs). At least for production and disposal, their entry into the environment is rather localised, e.g. through landfill leachates. This applies also to many other problematic contaminants. Cyanobacterial blooms occur at known water reservoirs, the major pathway of agrochemicals is in fact their entry through drainage systems (Schönenberger et al., 2022), and the majority of the most persistent pharmaceuticals, e.g. radio contrast agents, is released with hospital wastewaters. This suggests that the decentralised treatment at the respective hotspots is a more promising approach than the processing of large and diluted volumes in communal wastewater or drinking water plants. Therefore, however, a suitable technology is needed, which ideally can be operated autonomously, with little to no maintenance and without the need of consumables and complex infrastructures or support.

MODERN WATER TREATMENT OPTIONS

Regardless, water treatment plant operators in particular have responded to the new requirements that are imposed by the described challenges and the associated regulations. Their first choice was to rely on already established technologies that could be adopted from other fields and are readily available for the treatment of large volumes. Foremost, this has led to a more widespread use of biofilters, which, until recently, were considered the most advanced stage in most plants. In this case, microorganisms metabolise biodegradable organic compounds. The caveat is that many substances of concern, e.g. many pharmaceuticals or perfluorinated carbons, are not biodegradable. Furthermore, the operation requires expert experience and a sufficient control or at least adjustment of the operating parameters, such as ambient temperatures. Another promising approach is the introduction of ozonation in wastewater treatment plants based on the experience with this technology from drinking water supplies. The oxidising agents readily attack especially microorganisms and other pollutants and can successfully diminish the concentration of some problematic contaminants. Unfortunately, the oxidising potential of ozone is not sufficient to decompose many of the more interesting, i.e. more stable, compounds. Therefore, the method seems particularly promising to reduce the load of antibiotic resistant microorganisms. (This is also the main benefit of ozonation in drinking water treatment.) However, these conceivably already had ample opportunity to spread into the environment before they reached the wastewater treatment plant. Ultrafiltration and activated carbon filters are another means that were adopted from drinking water or exhaust gas treatment. Pollutants are retained or adsorbed by the filters, and with activated carbon in some cases even reduced. While successful in the original areas of application, the microorganisms that are always present in larger quantities in wastewater are prone to form biofilms on the filter material, which results in a rapid loss of their function. Moreover, the method is less effective for smaller and/or polar molecules. But even if pollutants are removed from the water, they are only physically retained on the filters. In addition to biofouling, this necessitates frequent backwashing and the subsequent treatment or disposal of the highly concentrated retentate and, in the case of activated carbon filters, eventually requires the disposal or regeneration of the filter material due to the accumulation of harmful substances. Because of the biofilm formation and the concentration of contaminants, the maintenance and replacement intervals are rather short and are associated with significant auxiliary costs. Another method, which was adopted from drinking water for wastewater treatment, is the exposure to ultraviolet light. By itself, only microorganisms are affected by the treatment, but the conversion of any chemicals is the rare exception. (Pollutants, which could be addressed this way, are also rather unstable and unproblematic since they would already have been decomposed by the exposure to sunlight.) The remediation of microorganisms exploits the inflicted damage to the genetic material of the cells. Moreover, the approach requires a low turbidity of the water for the light to penetrate deep into the volume, i.e. the clarification of wastewater to a sufficient degree. In summary, the thus far described technologies are not likely to provide a comprehensive solution for the removal of most of the persistent anthropogenic pollutants. Ozonation alone has shown an adequate degradation, at least of some pharmaceuticals, e.g. less stable antibiotics, and of cyanotoxins (Iakovides et al., 2019; Rodríguez et al., 2007). The latter is primarily a potential threat for drinking water, where the method has already been successfully established. The main advantage for all of the approaches is, however, that the respective systems and processes for the treatment of large volumes of water can already be supplied by the industry and the costs for installation and operation are well known, allowing for a detailed financial planning. Therefore, they have presumably been the methods of choice for many water treatment plants to address the requirements that have been imposed by European and national regulations. Accordingly, different pilot projects have been or are currently investigating their potential with substantial investment in the upgrading of facilities (Jekel, Altmann, et al., 2016; Jekel, Baur, et al., 2016; Kårelid et al., 2017; Meinel et al., 2014; Östman et al., 2019; Ullberg et al., 2021). Conversely, this strategy has probably hampered the further development of alternatives, which are more promising but are not yet at the same technological readiness level.

ADVANCED OXIDATION PROCESSES FOR WATER TREATMENT

Respective alternatives for water treatment are often described as advanced oxidation processes (AOPs). The principle operation of most concepts is based on the formation of hydroxyl radicals. With their high oxidation potential, these are able to oxidise and decompose almost every molecular structure. However, the radical is short-lived and is available for less than a microsecond as a reaction partner. Otherwise, it will react with itself or water for the formation of hydrogen peroxide, ozone (both still potent oxidising agents on their own), or eventually water and molecular oxygen. This requires the continuous and *in situ* generation of hydroxyl radicals in the treatment volume. Among the different possibilities, one of the more extensively investigated methods primarily relies on the cleavage of water when exposed to intense ultraviolet light. The radical production can be enhanced by adding hydrogen peroxide to the water. A further increase in efficiencies is achieved in contact with a photoactive semiconductor, e.g. titanium dioxide. Water and hydrogen peroxide can be oxidised to hydroxyl radicals when this catalyst is excited by ultraviolet light. The rather efficient process suffers again from the limitations of the penetration of light in turbid wastewaters. Photocatalysis using dispersed micro- or nanoparticles has been the most studied approach so far. However, the catalytic particles are an additional burden to the environment, i.e. pollutant. Their removal is often considered more cumbersome and costly than the originally intended water treatment itself. Other AOPs rely on Fenton's reaction, e.g. by combining iron salts with hydrogen peroxide, favour electrochemical water cleavage, albeit with relatively high currents, or even exploit a sonochemical generation of hydroxyl radicals. In most of these approaches, either hydrogen peroxide, ozone, or both are introduced into water, in addition, to increase the hydroxyl radical yield (Oturan & Aaron, 2014). A second look at the different methods, hence, reveals that either additional supplies are necessary, that the water has to be 'pre-conditioned'– e.g. with respect to conductivity, turbidity, or acidity, or that the treatment leaves other unwanted residuals – e.g. heterogeneous catalysts or sludge, which have to be addressed. Nevertheless, the mere potential thrives in ongoing investigations, in part already in relevant environments and settings (Miklos et al., 2018).

COLD PLASMA AS A WATER TREATMENT SOLUTION

Cold, or non-thermal, physical plasmas are another concept for the *in situ* generation of hydroxyl radicals, in particular, and reactive chemical species, in general. Their distinct advantage is that different approaches for an implementation do not require any consumables, including ozone or hydrogen peroxide. Instead, the plasma is realised with electrical discharges in the air or water directly and, therefore, only requires a suitable power supply. These inherent advantages of the technology are not accounted for when the comparison with other AOPs is based only on electrical energy efficiency, e.g. E_{EO}-values. Even within these constraints, cold plasma has established itself as a competitive alternative (Foster, 2017; Jiang et al., 2014).

In physics, plasma is frequently termed the 4th state of matter after solids, liquids, and gases in semblance to the phase transitions from one to the other. An illustrative example is the melting of ice to water and vaporisation of water to vapour. When the ice is heated, the strong and rigid bonds between the molecules are disrupted, and water molecules in the liquid can move against each other but are still attached to each other. In the gaseous state, the remaining interaction forces are discarded, and individual molecules can move independently from each other. If enough energy is supplied to the gas, eventually, electrons are excited and detached from atoms or molecules, leaving ions and excited species. These are highly reactive, as has already been described for hydroxyl radicals, and can form other potent reactive species, e.g. ozone, in subsequent reactions. In fact, the generation of ozone and ozonation is among the first plasma processes that have been studied in detail and applied as a disinfecting method. However, ozone generators are only one particular example for the successful implementation of plasma methods. In general, a large range of species can be produced that might actually offer more interesting alternatives for the treatment of water. But with more than 150 years of development, ozonation has matured to the current level as an obvious choice for many problems. Conversely, this success and history have probably impeded the further development and exploitation of other plasma processes for different applications, which, a century ago, probably did also look less feasible considering the available technical possibilities. With advances in power electronics, high voltages, which are the prerequisite for the generation of a plasma, can now be supplied in many different ways. This is the most important factor to establish different conditions and characteristics for a plasma with respect to specific discharge configurations. Especially for short high voltage pulses with a duration of only microseconds, or better yet nanoseconds, the associated energy is primarily transferred to electrons, which are the essence of the plasma. More abundant and energetic electrons will provide higher concentrations of the reactive species that are relevant for pollutant degradation. In comparison, the much heavier ions will not be able to significantly increase their kinetic energies. (An electron is about 2,000 times lighter than even the smallest ion, i.e. positively charged hydrogen. In an electric field, which is established through the application of a voltage, an electron can be more effectively accelerated, corresponding to the mass difference.) The latter determines the actual temperature of the reactive gaseous mixture of electrons and heavier species. Accordingly, the plasma is described as cold or non-thermal.

The high voltage needs to be applied between at least two electrodes for the generation of a plasma. This straightforward approach is also used in ozone generators where one extended electrode, e.g. a rod or wire, is surrounded by a tube, i.e. the other electrode. Other technical parameters for this coaxial arrangement, e.g. length of and distance between the electrodes, are foremost determined by the volumes that have to be treated and the power source that is needed to fill this volume with a plasma. In an ozone generator, the operating medium is a gas, i.e. air or oxygen. Accordingly, the plasma itself is not directly employed for the disinfection, which instead depends on the effluents, i.e. ozone, from the plasma. Arguably, more potent but short-lived species are not exploited by this indirect treatment. Therefore, research and development have focused on the possibilities to directly apply plasma to contaminated media, including water. Different configurations have been proposed and studied, which, in the best case, already consider the requirements for an effective treatment of water in terms of volumes and flow rates. Some of these are depicted in Figure 1.

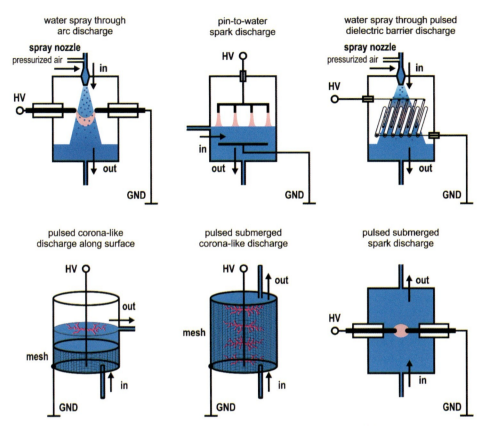

Figure 1. Concepts for the generation of cold plasma for water treatment. Reactive species, which are generated by the plasma, have to be effectively transported to pollutants by promoting the interaction between plasma and water.

The crucial factor for the degradation of pollutants is an optimisation of the interaction of the plasma with water. Therefore, the plasma is operated either in proximity to the liquid, for example by water sprays through the plasma, which, in this case can still be operated in gases, preferably ambient air. Accordingly, established methods and concepts can be adopted. These include arc and spark discharges or dielectric barrier discharges (DBDs). DBDs can be scaled to rather large areas with technologies and equipment that are already known for surface treatments. A way to increase the treatment area for spark discharges is by segmentation of the high voltage electrode or configurations with multiple electrodes. Another advantage of these concepts is the deliberate exploitation of plasma-chemical processes also with the constituents of air, i.e. oxygen and nitrogen, in addition to water. The respective reactive oxygen species (ROS) and reactive nitrogen species (RNS) have been identified as effective, especially as antimicrobial agents, but are also able to react with organic molecules, such as pharmaceuticals. A variation of discharges close to water are pulsed corona-like discharges. Both settings are interesting, in particular for pollutants, which accumulate at the surface, including perfluorinated carbons but also some agrochemicals, such as glyphosate. The concept of corona-like discharges can also be applied directly in the liquid. This is arguably the most efficient configuration for the generation of hydroxyl radicals by a plasma. The overall active plasma volume, which can be provided by this approach, is also primarily limited by the available power supplies. An additional benefit of this configuration is the simultaneously provided strong electric fields, which are an efficient means for the inactivation of microorganisms, e.g. *legionella*. Upon closer examination, it also becomes obvious that this concept is actually a transfer of the technology used for ozone generators into the liquid phase. In comparison, the treatment volume for submerged spark discharges is rather limited. Their main additional contribution to water treatments is strong shockwaves that are generated in addition to reactive chemical species. These are of interest for contaminants that should and could be broken up mechanically, e.g. algae.

All systems fulfill the requirement of the efficient production of reactive species and their effective transfer into the liquid. Which species are supplied, their production rates, and concentrations depend on particular underlying operating principles. Basically, spark, dielectric barrier, and corona-like discharges can be distinguished from each other and offer distinct advantages for specific pollutants. If hydroxyl radicals are needed, the submerged corona-like discharge seems to be the most appealing approach. However, the radical might not be necessary, for example, if cyanobacteria and cyanotoxins are addressed. In this case, the generation of RNS might be the economically preferred strategy. Consequently, non-thermal plasmas in general offer the flexibility to address certain problems with customised solutions. Since short-lived species are particularly responsible for the decomposition of pollutants, another unique characteristic of plasmas is that no explicitly harmful or toxic residues persist in the water after treatment. Eventually, even ozone or hydrogen peroxide is readily decomposed to water and oxygen under ambient conditions. Alone due to significant contributions of nitrogen to the operation could elevate nitrate- and nitrite-concentrations, which have to be addressed. In comparison, these are not relevant for submerged corona-like discharges.

DEGRADATION OF RECALCITRANT POLLUTANTS BY COLD PLASMA

Considering the possibilities, the increasing interest in non-thermal plasma and related research is not surprising. The degradation of numerous different pollutants that are considered a problem for water treatment has been demonstrated. This includes the degradation of pharmaceutical residues. In particular submerged corona-like discharges were successful in the almost complete decomposition of diclofenac and 17α-ethinylestradiol (Figure 2), which are considered substances of particular concern by the European Commission (Banaschik et al., 2015; European Parliament and Council of the European Union, 2013). Furthermore, the successful decomposition of agrochemicals, including a neonicotinoid that was also listed on the EU watchlist, by a water spray through a pulsed dielectric barrier discharge could also be shown as well as the decomposition of glyphosate with a pulsed corona-like discharge along a water surface (Zocher et al., 2021). Other compounds that could be addressed were bisphenol-A (Yang et al., 2022) or perfluorinated carbons (Singh et al., 2019), which also came into the focus of the European Commission (European Parliament and Council of the European Union, 2020). For the latter, a pin-to-water spark discharge was actually found to be the most efficient approach in comparison to other methods, such as electrochemical treatment, sonolysis, and activated persulfate (Singh et al., 2019). Also mycotoxins and cyanotoxins were decomposed by different electrical discharge configurations (Schneider et al., 2020; Wielogorska et al., 2019). That the potential of plasma-based water treatment is not only limited to the remediation of chemical pollutants but also offers advantages for a more traditional disinfection is visible through the inactivation of antibiotic resistant microorganisms in hospital wastewater by >99.9% and a complete inactivation, corresponding to a reduction by >99.999%, even for *legionella pneumophila* in a laboratory setting (Banaschik et al., 2016). In this case, the contribution of reactive species that were produced by a submerged corona-like discharge significantly enhances the effect of pulsed electric fields.

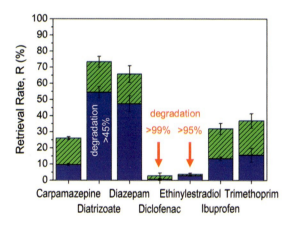

Figure 2. Retrieval rates for the treatment of different pharmaceuticals that were dissolved in water by submerged corona-like discharges. Especially diclofenac and ethinylestradiol could be almost completely decomposed. The method was also more successful than other approaches, e.g. ultraviolet light or ozonation, for the degradation of the radio contrast agent diatrizoate.

In part, studies have uncovered detailed decomposition pathways (Banaschik et al., 2018; Banaschik et al., 2017). In addition, several pilot-studies could already demonstrate economic viability as well (Ajo et al., 2018). Regardless, acceptance by the industry and water treatment plant operators is still limited. They would rather install matured systems for the treatment of large volumes of water, which are not available so far. The way towards such systems has been shown for ozone generators. However, research institutes do not have the means for such a product development. The situation could be improved by a change in funding strategies, i.e. if they would expand the current strong emphasis on the characterisation of water bodies and wastewater effluents towards methods for the remediation of pollutants. This would probably increase the interest of the industry to participate in activities and to contribute with their expertise.

Instead of the currently preferred implementation of the technology as the 4th stage in communal wastewater treatment plants, the more interesting application of the technology is probably found in decentralised systems at hotspots. The problematic pollutants that have been described are often released into the environment from point sources. For example, pharmaceutical residues in hospital wastewaters, perfluorinated carbons in the leachates of airports (as a result of their previous use in fire extinguishing foam), or drinking water reservoirs that are prone to cyanobacterial blooms. The list of potential applications could easily be expanded to include aquacultures (to reduce their need for freshwater intake), laundry services, and other enterprises with wastewaters with specific water pollutants from production or processing (e.g. food industry). Especially smaller companies cannot usually afford wastewater treatment systems and instead have to pay overcharges on their sewage disposals. However, once arriving at communal wastewater plants, the dilution and mixing with other contaminants poses a much greater problem for the treatment. However, an introduction of wastewater treatment for (small) companies would probably have to be supported or at least encouraged by regulation and legislation.

Local problems and a water treatment by decentralised units would directly play to the specific strengths of the technology, which is a sole requirement for electrical energy. Renewable energy sources, such as wind and sunlight, seem an obvious choice and are in good agreement with the goals of sustainability and environmental protection.

REFERENCES

Ajo, P., Preis, S., Vornamo, T., Mänttäri, M., Kallioinen, M., & Louhi-Kultanen, M. (2018). Hospital wastewater treatment with pilot-scale pulsed corona discharge for removal of pharmaceutical residues. *Journal of Environmental Chemical Engineering, 6*(2), 1569-1577. https://doi.org/https://doi.org/10.1016/j.jece.2018.02.007

Banaschik, R., Burchhardt, G., Zocher, K., Hammerschmidt, S., Kolb, J. F., & Weltmann, K. D. (2016). Comparison of pulsed corona plasma and pulsed electric fields for the decontamination of water containing Legionella pneumophila as model organism [Comparative Study]. *Bioelectrochemistry, 112*, 83-90. https://doi.org/10.1016/j.bioelechem.2016.05.006

Banaschik, R., Jablonowski, H., Bednarski, P. J., & Kolb, J. F. (2018). Degradation and intermediates of diclofenac as instructive example for decomposition of recalcitrant pharmaceuticals by hydroxyl radicals generated with pulsed corona plasma in water. *Journal of Hazardous Materials, 342*, 651-660. https://doi.org/10.1016/J.JHAZMAT.2017.08.058

Banaschik, R., Lukes, P., Jablonowski, H., Hammer, M. U., Weltmann, K. D., & Kolb, J. F. (2015). Potential of pulsed corona discharges generated in water for the degradation of persistent pharmaceutical residues [Research Support, Non-U.S. Gov't]. *Water Research, 84*, 127-135. https://doi.org/10.1016/j.watres.2015.07.018 Banaschik, R., Lukes, P., Miron, C., Banaschik, R., Pipa, A. V., Fricke, K., Bednarski, P. J., & Kolb, J. F. (2017). Fenton chemistry promoted by sub-microsecond pulsed corona plasmas for organic micropollutant degradation in water. *Electrochimica Acta, 245*, 539-548. https://doi.org/10.1016/j.electacta.2017.05.121

Brodin, T., Fick, J., Jonsson, M., & Klaminder, J. (2013). Dilute Concentrations of a Psychiatric Drug Alter Behavior of Fish from Natural Populations. *Science, 339*(6121), 814-815. https://doi.org/doi:10.1126/science.1226850

de Souza, R. M., Seibert, D., Quesada, H. B., de Jesus Bassetti, F., Fagundes-Klen, M. R., & Bergamasco, R. (2020). Occurrence, impacts and general aspects of pesticides in surface water: A review. *Process Safety and Environmental Protection, 135*, 22-37. https://doi.org/https://doi.org/10.1016/j.psep.2019.12.035

Devi, P. I., Manjula, M., & Bhavani, R. V. (2022). Agrochemicals, Environment, and Human Health. *Annual Review of Environment and Resources, 47*(1). https://doi.org/10.1146/annurev-environ-120920-111015

European Commission. (2022). Proposal for a Regulation of the European Parliament and of the Council on the sustainable use of plant proitection products and amending Regulation (EU) 2021/2115. https://eur-lex.europa.eu/legal-content/EN/TXT/?uri=COM%3A2022%3A305%3AFIN&qid=1656362428549

European Parliament and Council of the European Union. (2013). Directive 2013/39/

EU of the European Parliament and of the Council of 12 August 2013 amending Directives 2000/60/EC and 2008/105/EC as regards priority substances in the field of water policy. http://data.europa.eu/eli/dir/2013/39/oj

European Parliament and Council of the European Union. (2020). Directive (EU) 2020/2184 of the European Parliament and of the Council of 16 December 2020 on the quality of water intended for human consumption (recast). http://data.europa.eu/eli/dir/2020/2184/oj

Foster, J. E. (2017). Plasma-based water purification: Challenges and prospects for the future. *Physics of Plasmas, 24*(5). https://doi.org/10.1063/1.4977921

Hansen, H. C. B., Hilscherova, K., & Bucheli, T. D. (2021). Natural toxins: environmental contaminants calling for attention. *Environmental Sciences Europe, 33*(112). https://doi.org/10.1186/s12302-021-00543-6

Iakovides, I. C., Michael-Kordatou, I., Moreira, N. F. F., Ribeiro, A. R., Fernandes, T., Pereira, M. F. R., Nunes, O. C., Manaia, C. M., Silva, A. M. T., & Fatta-Kassinos, D. (2019). Continuous ozonation of urban wastewater: Removal of antibiotics, antibiotic-resistant Escherichia coli and antibiotic resistance genes and phytotoxicity. *Water Research, 159*, 333-347. https://doi.org/https://doi.org/10.1016/j.watres.2019.05.025

Jekel, M., Altmann, J., Ruhl, A. S., Sperlich, A., Schaller, J., Gnirß, R., Miehe, U., Stapf, M., Remy, C., & Mutz, D. (2016). *Integration der Spurenstoffentfernung in Technologieansätze der 4. Reinigungsstufe bei Klärwerken*. Universitätsverlag der TU Berlin. https://doi.org/10.14279/depositonce-4942

Jekel, M., Baur, N., Böckelmann, U., Dünnbier, U., Eckhardt, A., Gnirß, R., Grummt, T., Hummelt, D., Lucke, T., Meinel, F., Miehe, U., Mutz, D., Pflugmacher Lima, S., Reemtsma, T., Remy, C., Schlittenbauer, L., Schulz, W., Seiwert, B., Sperlich, A., . . . Ruhl, A. S. (2016). *Anthropogene Spurenstoffe und Krankheitserreger im urbanen Wasserkreislauf – Bewertung, Barrieren und Risikokommunikation (ASKURIS)*. Universitätsverlag der TU Berlin. https://doi.org/10.14279/depositonce-4979

Jiang, B., Zheng, J., Qiu, S., Wu, M., Zhang, Q., Yan, Z., & Xue, Q. (2014). Review on electrical discharge plasma technology for wastewater remediation. *Chemical Engineering Journal, 236*, 348-368. https://doi.org/https://doi.org/10.1016/j.cej.2013.09.090

Jönsson, J., Camm, R., & Hall, T. (2013). Removal and degradation of glyphosate in water treatment: a review. *Journal of Water Supply: Research and Technology-Aqua, 62*(7), 395-408. https://doi.org/10.2166/aqua.2013.080

Kårelid, V., Larsson, G., & Björlenius, B. (2017). Pilot-scale removal of pharmaceuticals in municipal wastewater: Comparison of granular and powdered activated carbon treatment at three wastewater treatment plants. *Journal of Environmental Management, 193*, 491-502. https://doi.org/https://doi.org/10.1016/j.jenvman.2017.02.042

Kim, K.-H., Kabir, E., & Jahan, S. A. (2017). Exposure to pesticides and the associated human health effects. *Science of The Total Environment, 575*, 525-535. https://doi.org/ https://doi.org/10.1016/j.scitotenv.2016.09.009

Meinel, F., Ruhl, A. S., Sperlich, A., Zietzschmann, F., & Jekel, M. (2014). Pilot-Scale Investigation of Micropollutant Removal with Granular and Powdered Activated Carbon. *Water, Air, & Soil Pollution, 226*(1), 2260. https://doi.org/10.1007/s11270-014-2260-y

Miklos, D. B., Remy, C., Jekel, M., Linden, K. G., Drewes, J. E., & Hübner, U. (2018). Evaluation of advanced oxidation processes for water and wastewater treatment – A critical review. *Water Research, 139*, 118-131. https://doi.org/10.1016/J. WATRES.2018.03.042

Monteiro, S. C., & Boxall, A. B. A. (2010). Occurrence and Fate of Human Pharmaceuticals in the Environment. In D. M. Whitacre (Ed.), *Reviews of Environmental Contamination and Toxicology* (pp. 53-154). Springer, New York. https://doi.org/10.1007/978-1-4419-1157-5_2

Östman, M., Björlenius, B., Fick, J., & Tysklind, M. (2019). Effect of full-scale ozonation and pilot-scale granular activated carbon on the removal of biocides, antimycotics and antibiotics in a sewage treatment plant. *Science of The Total Environment, 649*, 1117-1123. https://doi.org/https://doi.org/10.1016/j.scitotenv.2018.08.382

Oturan, M. A., & Aaron, J. J. (2014). Advanced Oxidation Processes in Water/Wastewater Treatment: Principles and Applications. A Review. *Critical Reviews in Environmental Science and Technology, 44*(23), 2577-2641. https://doi.org/10.1080/10643389.2013.8 29765

Purdom, C. E., Hardiman, P. A., Bye, V. V. J., Eno, N. C., Tyler, C. R., & Sumpter, J. P. (1994). Estrogenic Effects of Effluents from Sewage Treatment Works. *Chemistry and Ecology, 8*(4), 275-285. https://doi.org/10.1080/02757549408038554

Rodríguez, E., Onstad, G. D., Kull, T. P. J., Metcalf, J. S., Acero, J. L., & von Gunten, U. (2007). Oxidative elimination of cyanotoxins: Comparison of ozone, chlorine, chlorine dioxide and permanganate. *Water Research, 41*, 3381-3393. https://doi.org/10.1016/J. WATRES.2007.03.033

Schneider, M., & Bláha, L. (2020). Advanced oxidation processes for the removal of cyanobacterial toxins from drinking water. *Environmental Sciences Europe, 32*, 94. https://doi.org/10.1186/s12302-020-00371-0

Schneider, M., Rataj, R., Kolb, J. F., & Bláha, L. (2020). Cylindrospermopsin is effectively degraded in water by pulsed corona-like and dielectric barrier discharges. *Environmental Pollution, 266*. https://doi.org/https://doi.org/10.1016/j.envpol.2020.115423

Schönenberger, U. T., Simon, J., & Stamm, C. (2022). Are spray drift losses to agricultural roads more important for surface water contamination than direct drift to surface waters? *Science of The Total Environment, 809*, 151102. https://doi.org/https://doi. org/10.1016/j.scitotenv.2021.151102

Singh, R. K., Multari, N., Nau-Hix, C., Anderson, R. H., Richardson, S. D., Holsen, T. M., & Mededovic Thagard, S. (2019). Rapid Removal of Poly- and Perfluorinated Compounds from Investigation-Derived Waste (IDW) in a Pilot-Scale Plasma Reactor. *Environmental Science & Technology, 53*(19), 11375-11382. https://doi.org/10.1021/acs.est.9b02964

Stackelberg, P. E., Furlong, E. T., Meyer, M. T., Zaugg, S. D., Henderson, A. K., & Reissman, D. B. (2004). Persistence of pharmaceutical compounds and other organic wastewater contaminants in a conventional drinking-water-treatment plant [Research Support, U.S. Gov't, P.H.S.]. *The Science of the total environment, 329*(1-3), 99-113. https://doi.org/10.1016/j.scitotenv.2004.03.015

Ternes, T. A., Meisenheimer, M., McDowell, D., Sacher, F., Brauch, H. J., Gulde, B. H., Preuss, G., Wilme, U., & Seibert, N. Z. (2002). Removal of pharmaceuticals during drinking water treatment. *Environmental Science & Technology, 36*(17), 3855-3863. https://doi.org/10.1021/es015757k

Ullberg, M., Lavonen, E., Köhler, S. J., Golovko, O., & Wiberg, K. (2021). Pilot-scale removal of organic micropollutants and natural organic matter from drinking water using ozonation followed by granular activated carbon [10.1039/D0EW00933D]. *Environmental Science: Water Research & Technology, 7*(3), 535-548. https://doi.org/10.1039/D0EW00933D

Wielogorska, E., Ahmed, Y., Meneely, J., Graham, W. G., Elliott, C. T., & Gilmore, B. F. (2019). A holistic study to understand the detoxification of mycotoxins in maize and impact on its molecular integrity using cold atmospheric plasma treatment. *Food Chemistry, 301*, 125281. https://doi.org/https://doi.org/10.1016/j.foodchem.2019.125281

Yang, J., Zeng, D., Hassan, M., Ma, Z., Dong, L., Xie, Y., & He, Y. (2022). Efficient degradation of Bisphenol A by dielectric barrier discharge non-thermal plasma: Performance, degradation pathways and mechanistic consideration. *Chemosphere, 286*, 131627.

Zocher, K., Gros, P., Werneburg, M., Brser, V., Kolb, J. F., & Leinweber, P. (2021). Degradation of glyphosate in water by the application of surface-corona-discharges. *Water Science and Technology, 84*(5), 1293-1301. https://doi.org/10.2166/wst.2021.320

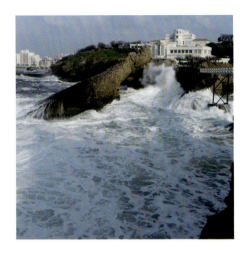
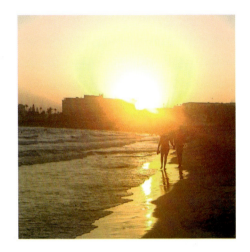
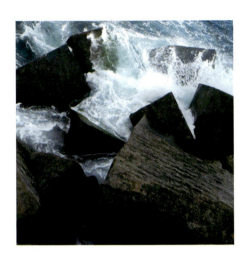
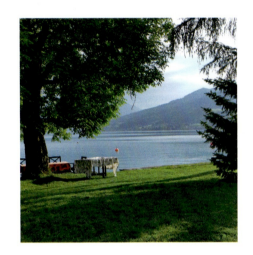
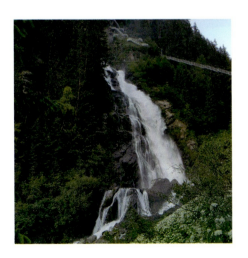
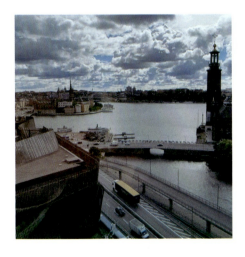

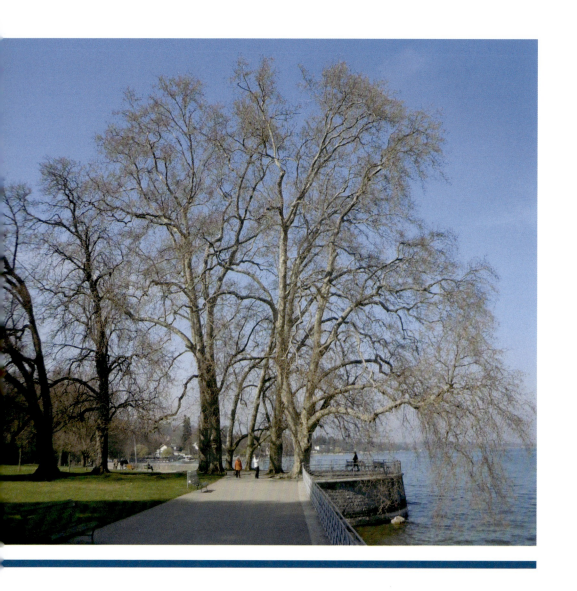

INNOVATION AND DELAY
IN SMART MEASURING DEVICES
FOR WATER SYSTEMS

Armando Di Nardo (Università della Campania Luigi Vanvitelli, Med.Hydro company), Anna Di Mauro (Med.Hydro company), Jordi Cros (Med.Hydro company, ADASA company)

The spread of Information and Communication Technologies (ICT), digital technologies, and new monitoring systems in the last decade has overcome a key factor in the water-smart society. This great evolution is based on of digitalisation of data, which converts it into information and later on in knowledge. Digitisation allows for a very useful and innovative data management and control, specifically summarised in: store information; stream / send / share information without noise or errors; add additional multi-dimensional information (time, location, ...) for further processing; treat and process the information to control, analyse, predict, etc.; implementation of IoT, BigData, Machine Learning, Artificial Intelligence, etc. techniques.

A Smart Measurement Device (SMD) is a set of necessary elements thanks to the signal supplied by the sensors, which in relation to the parameter that must be converted to a digital representation, provides the measurement in the appropriate format. This process can be simple (just convert an analogue voltage to a digital value and multiply it by a factor to obtain the parameter) or complex, for example some processes, reagents and complex mathematical operations are needed to obtain the desired parameter. ICT technologies are related with smart measuring devices as they are the basis of the digitalisation and processing of measurements.

As investigated in the Working Group of Water Europe WATERSET (WATER Sensors and Tools), composed by different and qualified stakeholders as water utilities; research centres and universities; large, medium, and small companies and operators; and, as appropriately, reported in many scientific and technical papers, more problems in terms of gaps, barriers, shortcomings, etc. are present and are identifiable to a full application of SMD on the market of water distribution networks.

In this short document, a more extensive version will be published by Water Europe as a white paper recommendation for the European Union, the main issues are exposed with reference to gaps, delays, and some possible solutions.

The Smart Measuring Devices allow monitoring water quantity and quality parameters with reference to the physical, chemical, and biological categories of measurements, and whether they are accessible locally or remotely. But characteristics of these categories affect the measuring device, because to convert an analogue representation (measurement parameter) into a digital representation, the signals provided by sensors must be electrical signals (voltage / current), by comparison with reference, and digital signals (Frequency / Time), by counting.

The different parameters supplied by Smart Measuring Devices are:

a) Physical parameters (quantity & quality) (e.g. level, flow, temperature, conductivity): easy and simple conversion of measured parameter into a digitizable signal; the measuring device is near the sensor; the devices are stable over time, they do not have excessive wear, they need little calibration.

b) Chemical parameters (Quality) (pH, RedOx, free chlorine, nutrients, ions, ...): a conversion to a physical parameter must be carried out; the measurement device can be complex, as the sensor can work only under certain conditions, so it often requires reagents; not stable over time and usually requires calibration (the conversion from chemical to physical parameters usually produces "wear").

c) Biological parameters (Quality) (BDO5, toxicity, microbiological indicators, ...): it is necessary to carry out a conversion to physical parameters; the measuring device is usually very complex and often requires reagents; if the conversion of the biological parameter is through an intermediate step of a chemical parameter, as the process of conversion from chemical to physical parameter usually produces "wear", they are not stable over time and may need calibration.

Smart Measuring Devices for water are expected to foster innovation across the Water Value Chain (WVC). In the water sector, innovative meters – able to measure diffusely quantity and quality parameters with low capital and operational costs, low energy consumption, and cloud connections – can allow identifying novel solutions able to face the socio-economic challenges of water use, water quality, and management according to various stakeholders' operational needs. The integration of analysers, smart meters, and biosensors with cloud computing and innovative Big Data analytics and machine learning approaches allows for the improve of network management and to align the water sector with other public utility sectors like energy and telecommunications.

The expected ideal characteristics that Smart Measuring Devices should have are:

- small size in order to be spread out as "dust sensors;"
- low CAPEX (capital expenditure) and low OPEX (operational expenditure);
- easy to install;
- easy to collect and transmit information or data (connecting to a cloud);
- low energy consumption.

Then these SMD would allow for a wider dissemination into the water network, the possibility to be used as Big Data, Artificial Intelligence, and Machine Learning techniques, and the interpretation of alteration in quality and quantity measures to allow for the prediction of system behaviour also in the perspective of an early warning, and, more in general, to improve control of the water systems.

Anyway, it is clear that some gaps, barriers, and delays in the industrialisation and dissemination of SMD are still present to meet the paradigm of smart cities regarding different issues as technological, economic, legislative, and integration. Specifically, issues can be categorised into technological, economical, legislative, and integration.

In general, it is possible to state that, in the last twenty years, the evolution in sensors **technology** was low due to physical limits, while a great evolution in ICT of sensors was observed. Many measuring devices are just automated laboratory equipment and not yet able to be used in the wide disseminated area because of the high costs of purchasing and maintenance. Therefore, smart metering devices are still in an embryonic and experimental stage and are not yet commercially available.

Evidently, the crucial **economical** point is that, currently, smart sensors may be cheap, but smart analysers are not. In this way, it is not possible to imagine the wide dissemination of smart devices in the water distribution networks or in other segments managed by water utilities. So, there are high costs for the realisation, installation, commissioning, maintenance, and communications.

Indeed, actually in Europe, only laboratory measurements (no online or smart measuring devices) have been accepted in **legislation**, and the frequency of the required measurements is too low to need more performance devices and the application of big data and machine learning analysis. So, it is possible to state, without denial, that legislation does not promote the use of water quality smart measurement devices and represents the main barrier for the full development and dissemination of SMD in the water sector. The lack of specific guidelines and directive for the standardisation of the implementation and usage of devices and data recorded is clear.

Another issue regards the problem of the **integration** of SMD in design, management, and control policies of water utilities and operators because the possibility of having a large number of smart metering devices opens new operational and technical challenges as, for example: Where to install SMD to obtain optimal performance? Which direct and indirect parameters are more useful? With the help of SMD widely disseminated, is it possible to reduce the number of direct parameters to measure? Which are the optimal time-intervals to select in order to obtain enough information for big data analysis and machine learning procedures? Which tools and software are reliable and standardised? Therefore, there is the necessity together with the improvement of new technologies for smart metering, to develop new criteria, procedures, tools, and software for defining an integrated framework for the application of these new technologies in real context.

Therefore, some possible solutions and recommendations have been delineated to address the issues which arise during the survey conducted by WATERSET Working Group, and are reported in the following:

- **Technological**: it is mandatory to promote research and innovation projects to develop smart metering technologies. Thanks to the massive amount of recorded data, it becomes crucial to promote the use of artificial intelligence, big data analysis, and machine learning tools for data management in the water sector to better understand the system behaviour and to allow prediction and early warning.
- **Economic**: it is necessary to reach the market with the technologies that have already been validated in order to stimulate the creation of a volume market and assure the migration from research to market.
- **Legislation**, it is necessary to change the water monitoring legislation in terms of legal requirements for online monitoring, and data privacy and security, so it will be possible to reach the market with the technologies that have already been validated;
- **Integration issues**, it is also important to define guidelines for the employment of sensing systems in view of a unified standardisation.

These improvements can be possible only with the cooperation between the stakeholders, research groups, and national and community governments.

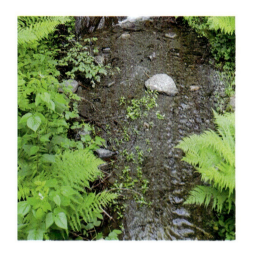
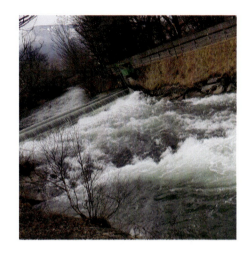
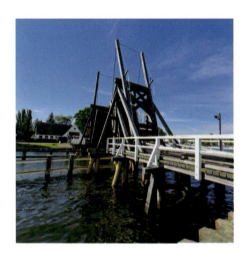
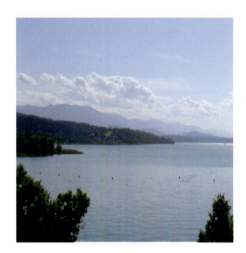
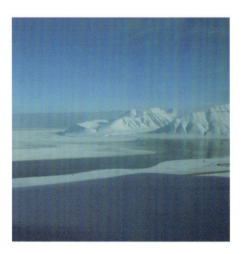
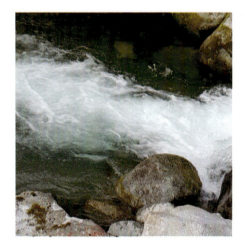

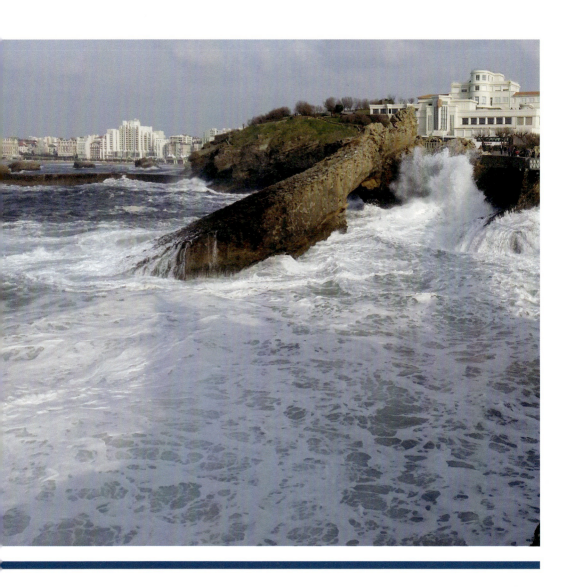

WATER DATA SPACE

CHALLENGES AND OPPORTUNITIES

Eloisa Vargiu (CETaqua, Water Technology Centre, Barcelona),
Roberto Di Bernardo (Engineering Ingegneria Informatica SpA, Rome),
Rafael Gimenez-Esteban (CETaqua, Water Technology Centre, Barcelona),
Davide Storelli (Engineering Ingegneria Informatica SpA, Rome)

ABSTRACT

The Digital Water Systems and Interoperability working group at Water Europe aims to contribute to the creation of a water data space in the context of the European data spaces by contributing to the relevant initiatives around data sharing and standardisation from a water data perspective; liaising with key entities in the area; encouraging the creation of project proposals in that direction, as well as disseminating reference implementations and APIs. This chapter briefly introduces the main challenges and opportunities to reaching this objective.

INTRODUCTION

The volume of data produced in the world is growing rapidly, from 33 zettabytes in 2018 to an expected 175 zettabytes in 2025[1]. Nowadays, 80% of the processing and analysis of data takes place in data centres and centralised computing facilities, while only 20% occurs in smart connected objects – such as cars, home appliances, or manufacturing robots, and in computing facilities close to the user. By 2025, these proportions are likely to be inverted[2], the EU Strategy for data will have been fully implemented, multiple data spaces will have been widely adopted across Europe, and European individuals and organisations will have regained the possibility of control over their data and their rightful and balanced place in the digital world. By 2030, it will be the mainstream scenario, and the larger audience will not accept it any other way[3].

When considering the creation of data spaces in Europe, it is important to highlight the alignment of key initiatives such as BDVA[4], FIWARE[5], GAIA-X[6], and IDSA[7]. FIWARE is bringing today mature technologies, compatible with the IDSA and GAIA-X envisioned global standard as well as specifications and interfaces for data sovereignty and sharing in line with the European research towards the implementation of data space (relevant here is the BDVA strategic research and innovation agenda). The four initiatives are now formally collaborating around DSBA[8], the alliance aiming at converging the best skills, assets, and experiences in Europe into a one-stop-shop for data spaces, from inception

---

1 https://www.idc.co.za/financial-results/2018-annual-report/
2 https://www.gartner.com/smarterwithgartner/2017-the-year-that-data-and-analytics-go-mainstream
3 Design principles for data spaces: https://design-principles-for-data-spaces.org/
4 Big Data Value Association: https://www.bdva.eu/
5 https://www.fiware.org/
6 https://gaia-x.eu/
7 International Data Spaces: https://internationaldataspaces.org
8 Data Space Business Alliance: https://data-spaces-business-alliance.eu/

to deployment, to accelerate business transformation in the data economy.

Among different domains, this chapter focuses on the challenges and opportunities of implementing and adopting data spaces in the water sector. After introducing the data space concept and main design principles, the specific water sector case is discussed.

DATA SPACES

A data space is defined as a decentralised infrastructure for trustworthy data sharing and exchange in data ecosystem based on commonly agreed principles. Following gathered stakeholders' concerns, the main design principles for data spaces has been derived: (i) data sovereignty, the capability of a natural person or corporate entity for exclusive self-determination regarding its economic data goods; (ii) data level playing field, implies that new entrants face no insurmountable barriers when seeking admission to a data space; (iii) decentralised soft infrastructure, which will be made of the totality of interoperable implementations of data spaces complying with a set of agreements in terms of functional, technical, operational, and legal aspects; and (iv) public-private governance, by promoting the broad adoption of European data spaces and building up and maintaining a development community.

WATER DATA SPACE

Motivation

The EU can become a leading role model for a society empowered by data to make better decisions – in business and the public sector. Cities and communities represent a fertile environment for effective innovation. To boost local ecosystems and enable the transition towards a data society, data spaces represent a key enabler of the Green Deal goals[9] and Sustainable Development Goals[10]. Nevertheless, to achieve the aforementioned goals, a systemic approach has to be followed by considering the so-called Key Community Systems, like water management.

Specifically for the water sector, digitalisation represents a key transformation factor, which can be leveraged to implement strategic policy commitments and directives at national, European, and international levels. It underpins a transformation process towards more resilient and sustainable water services and data-driven decisions, generating benefits for the society, the economy, and the environment by facilitating the optimisation of the resources' consumption, the enhancement of health and safety, as

---

9 https://ec.europa.eu/info/strategy/priorities-2019-2024/european-green-deal_en
10 https://sdgs.un.org/goals

well as the minimisation of negative socio/economic impacts due to climate change. It is thus fundamental to improve decision making and action planning by leveraging on the available data, despite whether such data is dispersed, non-standardised, and generally of low quality.

Challenges

According to the design principles defined for the data spaces, let us consider here some specific aspects regarding the water sector.

Data sovereignty. Water data sharing strategies between companies and countries are actually poorly implemented and require affordable and trustworthy data sovereignty and provenance mechanism. FIWARE delivers several components for creating data spaces, with particular emphasis on trust and data sovereignty following IDSA specifications. They aim at reducing the entry barriers and, thus, the cost of data sharing and exchange. This has also been achieved by creating a semantic standard for data sovereignty, i.e. the rules and policies that determine who is allowed to do what in which context with the data shared by the data owner.

Data level playing field. For the effective application of effective data management and data sharing in the water sector and for the ultimate success of water data spaces, societal integration is needed. Its success depends on social acceptance and consent of the benefits of the data spaces, irrespective of the technological achievements and their (current) degree of implementation. At the EU level, the ICT4WATER cluster[11] is promoting data sharing, interoperability, and standardisation towards the adoption of a reference architecture for data injection, accessibility, sharing, and consumption. This strategy falls under the transformation of the water sector towards the generation of data spaces that permit to interlink all water value chains with also cross-domain sectors.

Decentralised soft infrastructure. OpenDEI[3] presents and proposes a soft infrastructure for data spaces to build scalable, interoperable, and trustworthy solutions, which enables mass and sector-agnostic adoption and ensures that agreements and standards are aligned with the building blocks. The latter are categorised as interoperability, trust, data value, and governance. That soft infrastructure can also be simply applied and adopted for water data.

Public-private governance. Transnational public-private partnerships are new forms of governance that have caught the interest of researchers in recent years. Comparing and analysing the performance of three transnational water partnerships, Beisheim and Campe [1] showed that a high degree of institutionalisation tends to be important for those water partnerships that implement costly projects. It is less important for those that focus on the comparatively undemanding task of exchanging and disseminating knowledge and best practice in water management and governance. On the other hand,

---

11 https://ict4water.eu/

improving water data governance is the key to addressing water insecurity in developing countries. Araral and Wang [2] reviewed the literature on water governance and find that, first, there appears to be little consensus on the scope and definition of water governance. Second, while water governance is inherently multidisciplinary and interdisciplinary in nature, there is little evidence of this in the literature. Third, the literature is generally descriptive and argumentative and offers little theoretical coherence. As a main conclusion, they argued for a second-generation multidisciplinary research agenda on water governance, which integrates economics, politics, and administration, and also pays more attention to incentive issues and has clear policy implications.

Opportunities

Citizens should be empowered to make better decisions based on insights gleaned from data. Data should be available to all – whether public or private, big or small, start-up or giant. This will help society to get the most out of innovation and competition and ensure that everyone benefits from a digital dividend. On the other hand, citizens will trust and embrace data-driven innovations only if they are confident that any personal data sharing in the EU will be subject to full compliance with the EU's strict data protection rules. At the same time, the increasing volume of non-personal industrial data and public data in Europe – combined with technological change in how the data is stored, shared, and processed – will constitute a potential source of growth and innovation that should be tapped into.

New competences must be created/enforced around the exploitation of data driven business models in the water ecosystems. An actual barrier against data economy undertaken within the water sector is the missing perception of a concrete value out of it. Efforts (and related costs) to be spent to make own data sharable with other actors is still considered much too high in respect of the possible incomes transversally generated by new possible business opportunities (data enabled).

Digital Europe should reflect the best of Europe – open, fair, diverse, democratic, and confident. The water sector is undergoing a gradual digital transformation that is affecting the entire water lifecycle with a maturity level that varies from case to case: from simply incorporating sensors into operational procedures to capture relevant data, visualise trends and raise alerts about anomalous events to sophisticated AI-based approaches to data analysis to produce predictions/simulations and to support automated and optimised operations in the field. Under the perspective of data spaces, as the level of maturity raises, there is a big opportunity to merge and integrate data from different sources, pulling data-resources from other correlated sectors – including urban infrastructures, climate, and energy, in order to understand interdependencies and generate value-added insight about their nexus and their combined impact on society and on the environment, and thus actually implementing the systemic approach envisioned to meet the UN agenda goals.

CONCLUSION

Converging European approaches into a one-stop-shop for data spaces enables new business solutions in chosen domains as described in the European data strategy (energy, Green Deal, industry, public, finance, agriculture, skills, mobility) or even across domains, while the experimentation of data spaces increases. Eventually, while standardisation proceeds and more experience is gathered, the deployment rate of data spaces will increase through the adoption of scalable data spaces' building blocks. Focusing on the water sector, digitalisation represents a key transformation factor, which can make the difference for the implementation of strategic policy commitments and directives at national, European, and international levels.

In this chapter, we briefly addressed the main challenges and opportunities for a water data space. Challenges consist basically of (i) data sovereignty; (ii) data level playing field; (iii) decentralised soft infrastructure; and (iv) public-private governance. Opportunities will be seized only if a holistic approach is embraced and is capable to lead to effective digital transformation across multiple dimensions: (i) human, behavioural changes at the individual level require effective digital training of the workforce, possibly with life-long learning programmes to upskill digital professionals in the water sector; (ii) organisational, promoting data culture and multi-disciplinary collaboration; (iii) technological, extending the use of data-driven decision support systems that leverage state-of-the-art artificial intelligence and provide an integrated view of the cyber-physical system, ensuring high-level cybersecurity standards; (iv) data, data availability and quality – based on common standards for data sharing and interoperability – are fundamental enablers for unlocking opportunities in the new European era of "data" economy; and (v) governance, top-down (pressure of directives and polices) and bottom-up (common vision among stakeholders, convincing demonstration cases) approaches should be combined to develop innovative governance systems centred on the value of water (and on digital transformation as an enabler).

REFERENCES

[1] Beisheim, M. and Campe, S., 2012. Transnational public–private partnerships' performance in water governance: institutional design matters. Environment and Planning C: Government and Policy, 30(4), pp.627-642.

[2] Araral, E. and Wang, Y., 2013. Water governance 2.0: a review and second generation research agenda. Water Resources Management, 27(11), pp.3945-3957.

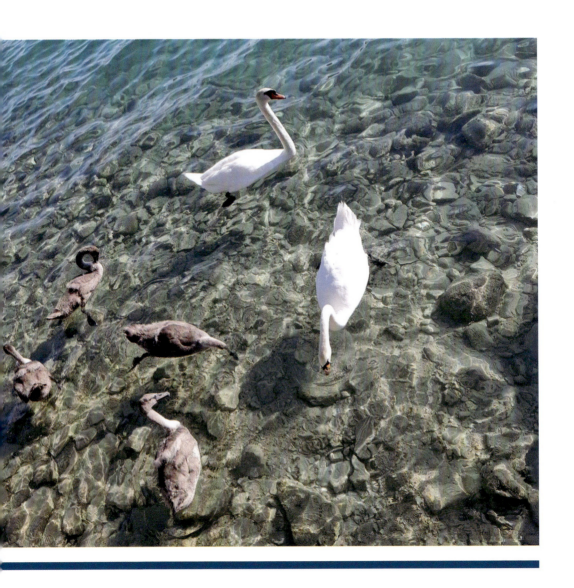

THE RELEVANCE OF HUMAN CAPITAL AS A DRIVING FORCE TOWARD AN INCLUSIVE WATER-SMART COMMUNITY

Naomi Timmer (Director H2O People B.V.),
Rasha Hassan (PhD candidate at the University of Barcelona,
Project officer at H2O-People B.V.)

INTRODUCTION

As we deal with major transformations and rapid changes in a complex world, we need to be able to adapt and change the frames we use to come to actionable solutions (Véricourt, Cukier, and Mayer-Schönberger 2021). The water community is at risk of disruption of automation and shocks such as COVID-19 through which 29% of the water supply and sewerage, 33% of public administration, 38% of the education sector will be impacted (Smit et al., 2020). In addition, there is a gap between policy and actions in the aforementioned topics with limitations across the value chain which hinder the transformations and forward thinking in the water sector (Timmer and Hassan 2022a).

Thus, the water sector – specifically decision-makers – needs a roadmap to find effective strategies and programmes to delineate future career paths, smooth these transitions, and solve the challenge of mismatches. Young water professionals represent a key force in setting the agenda for future transitions.

Following this idea, this is a crucial moment in which we can integrate the past, present, and future to establish a dynamic joint vision of the future workplace. This chapter reports on an intergenerational dialogue between different actors and representatives within the water sector which took place in the New Waves Festival "The Future of the Workplace in the European Sector."

METHODOLOGY

We opted to create an interactive setting to establish an efficient intergenerational dialogue and to provide a safe environment for exploring ideas and the actions needed for this transformation. The attendees came from different backgrounds and expertise levels within the water sector from which ca. 50% were part of the European Junior Water Programme. The co-creators were selected based on their expertise in theme, roles, and driving forces of transitions in their field.

THE FESTIVAL AS A CO-CREATION MODEL

The goal of the festival was to facilitate a co-creative space in which collaboration and creativity were used to achieve real results, not only for the content but also for the network and development. The transformation in the water sector was discussed in regard to different topics, and a co-creator was assigned to each one.

DEEP DEMOCRACY: THE COLLABORATIVE SKILLS DEVELOPMENT TOOL

Deep Democracy is a set of simple yet powerful tools and skills which was developed in South Africa by clinical psychologists Myrna and Greg Lewis (Lewis and Woodhull 2018; Myrna Lewis and Lewis 2018) and made adaptable for organisations by anthropologist Jitske Kramer in the Netherlands (Jitske Kramer, 2020). It is a cutting-edge facilitation and conflict transformation methodology that is pragmatic, easily acquired and can be used by people with no psychology training. As part of the Erasmus+ Strategic Partnership SMARTEN, we implement and support the digital acceleration by adopting such a tool to support augmented collaboration and inclusive conversations within the water sector (Timmer and Hassan 2022b).

RESULTS AND DISCUSSION

Let's look deeper into these topics and how they relate back to the major themes identified in an Open Space Approach Event at the New Waves Festival 2022 "The Future Workplace of European Water" (Timmer and Hassan 2022a) and what will happen with the necessary transformations and actions identified during the event.

DIGITALISATION AND AUTOMATION

We have seen an automation and digitalisation acceleration by the pandemic especially affecting those who were already at risk of being affected by automation if we look at replacement (Smith et al., 2020).The uptake of digital technology from the existing EU R&D&I has been weak and slow, and it is seen through the fragmented innovations in the water sector. It also lacks a robust preparation of future specialists who are ready to implement and utilise these innovations. This step should start from the university curricula orientation towards new priorities: holistic water ecosystem for the digitisation of the urban water sector, upgrading internet services in the water sector, protection of water infrastructure against cyber threats, etc. A joint effort from companies, academia, and government (triple helix) is required to facilitate the uptake of digital innovations in operational environments (Working Group Human Capital 2021). Stakeholders are not adequately involved/cooperative when seeking innovative digital solutions today. Therefore, improving the educational requirements to prepare future employees for the digitalising world is crucial along with a closer interaction among the tripe helix.

HAPPY AND HEALTHY WATER PEOPLE

There is a need to offer training and coaching for social and emotional skills to facilitate the growing focus on the interconnections within the water sector (Smith et al., 2020). This is highly needed due to the changes that the automation brings and from the technological perspective also creates more attention to what does make people special and needed in the workplace (Véricourt et al., 2021; Yang 2020). Especially when we look at the topic of innovation, we also see the input of the ICT sector and also of the influence of psychology and anthropology on this topic (Edmondson 2019; Kramer 2021). Their combined perspective on the added value of human beings in the workplace is to emphasise the power of the mindset, storytelling, and creating community, which creates meaning for the work. While Yang (2020) is looking for solutions in freedom thinking, people focused capitalism, people to people learning, to training how to live good, positive, and socially productive lives. Still remains the question: how can this be done well in a digital format? This is something that we need to find out.

What we come to terms with, and often tell young professionals that they need, is the feeling of mattering in their job. A job that gives meaning to why and for whom they are doing their work. They are then called idealists, but don't we all need to feel that what we do in life matters? Which frame or ideal we attach to this human urge doesn't matter, but it creates the importance for all individuals to feel seen and acknowledged and makes people happy and healthy. So that is also something to be taken into consideration when creating a healthy and happy workforce in water.

OUT OF OUR 'WATER' BUBBLE

To become ready for the future workplace, we need to face the discomfort of what and who is the water sector. The day before the New Waves Festival, one of Water Europe's Flagship Events, "Water Innovation Europe" (14-15 June 2022, Brussels), took place. During the event we heard quite often from very knowledgeable people that they are not 'water experts'. They knew, for example, a lot about international law and human rights or about politics and governance. Is that not part of water, too? Do we not need these people in the water sector? Just as we need ICT people to become water people as well? Don't we view 'the water sector' as too small and forget it is part of a holistic system? We need a more expansive definition of a water professional to tackle this but also to change the frame we're working in. The inclusion of new backgrounds is not only something nice, to be more diverse, but it also creates more knowledge, more potential people within the sector, and more innovation (Kramer 2021; Meyer 2019).

To get out of our water bubble we need to see what is not there yet but could and should be. We could do this by creating and trying new frames (Véricourt et al., 2021). It makes us understand the world and change it, and isn't that what we are trying to do when we create solutions for the water sector within a holistic approach? To do this we need to celebrate conflict and alternatives (Kramer 2021; Véricourt et al., 2021) and use the diversity of thinking, acting, and behaving from the different cultures around Europe. This collaboration across boundaries creates challenges, to understanding each other, but it can also be a source for continuous learning and experiences (Meyer 2019).

LEADERSHIP AND EMPOWERMENT

Neil Dhot (AquaFed) and Durk Krol (Water Europe) started their search during the New Waves Festival with the question what employers need to know from young professionals/ need to change to stay connected and transform (Timmer and Hassan 2022a). Smith et al. (2020) identified the challenges and priorities for employers per archetype of the workforce. Combining this with the outcomes of the festival, we mainly see a focus in the water sector from a perspective of high tech producers and high skilled white-collar workers with a priority of attracting (and retaining) (STEM) talent, promoting cultural lifelong learning, continuous improvement, agility, and innovation, and to enable the retraining and redeployment of existing workforce towards more productive tasks. Offering training and coaching for social and emotional skills to facilitate a growing focus on customer experience and client relationships (Smith et al., 2020).

A focus on these groups seems to be understandable, since in the future this will be the group with the biggest growth expectancy and also the largest shortage in personnel (Smith et al., 2020). The high average age level in the sector might also be beneficial, since a lot of the workers that are at risk of replacement due to automation will leave the sector automatically. One of the topics not being taken into consideration during the New Waves Festival is the knowledge transfer of these workers into the automation process as well as the skills to adapt to the changing circumstances.

From the side of European policymakers, the adaptation to green skills is highly encouraged as well as programmes to ensure diversity and sustainability in different sectors. An example, the SPIRE SAIS project, is a European supported Erasmus + Strategic Partnership to create a blueprint for a new learning and skill system for energy intensive industries to work on energy efficiency and industrial symbiosis from industry and skill providers' perspective.
The Valuing of Water Initiative from the Dutch Government and their focus within their youth programme on career path developments was presented at the New Waves Festival. Europe needs to create more training and career pathways and support partnerships between educators and employers in the design of the career-relevant curricula necessary to set up effective training, better job matching, and transition

support (Smith et al., 2020). Since acquired skills are changing rapidly, employers seem to be the natural providers of training opportunities, and policy makers should think of incentives to execute this with the best for the individual working in mind. Access to trainings outside of the workplace are therefore essential as well (Smith et al., 2020). Another important task for the policymakers is ensuring a healthy workplace framework within the combination between the virtual and local workplace.

Automation brings us to the transition where we need to work on "Masters or Slaves," so we need to empower ourselves to create a better world (Yang 2020). We cannot do that by becoming slaves of our time but take leadership and fight for it together.

To create a new frame for the workplace of the water sector we all need a new mindset (Véricourt et al., 2021). Therefore it was hopeful that in the action lists of the New Waves Festival those who had to get into action mainly pointed at ourselves (Timmer and Hassan 2022a).

CONCLUSION

In addition to the technical developments and transformations in the water sector, we need to invest resources in the human factor. A range of transformations impact this – shown from the experiences of practitioners throughout the value chain at the New Waves Festival and supported by literature. We need to work together with all different types of organisations and partners from without and now outside of the sector to build a better future. We need to redefine who we see as part of the water sector and make our community more diverse and holistic to be able to reach our common goal of enough clean water within the system for our lives as humans and the Earth, now and in the future.

REFERENCES

Edmondson, Amy. 2019. *The Fearless Organization: Creating Psychological Safety in the Workplace for Learning, Innovation, and Growth.* Gildan Media, LLC.

Kramer, Jitske. 2021. *Jam Cultures: Inclusion: Having a Seat at the Table, a Voice and a Vote: About Inclusion; Joining in the Action, Conversation and Decisions.* Management Impact.

Kramer, Jitske. 2020, *Deep Democracy: De wijsheid van de minderheid*, Management Impact.

Lewis, Myrna and Jennifer Woodhull. 2018. *Inside The NO: Five Steps to Decisions That Last.*

Meyer, Erin. 2014. *The Culture Map: Breaking Through the Invisible Boundaries of Global Business.*

Myrna Lewis and Greg Lewis. n.d. "Lewis Deep Democracy." Retrieved May 3, 2022 (https://www.lewisdeepdemocracy.com/).

Smit, Sven, Tilman Tacke, Susan Lund, James Manyika, and Lea Thiel. 2020. *The Future of Work in Europe: Automation, Workforce Transitions, and the Shifting Geography of Employment.*

Timmer, Naomi and Rasha Hassan. 2022a. *New Waves Festival 2022: The Future Workplace of European Water.*

Timmer, Naomi and Rasha Hassan. 2022b. "The Augmented Collaboration Toolkit."

Véricourt, Francis de, Kenneth Cukier, and Viktor Mayer-Schönberger. 2021. *Framers: Human Advantages in an Age of Technoloy and Turmoil.* Amsterdam: Maven Publishing.

Working Group Human Capital, Water Europe. 2021. *The Future Needs of Human Capital Development in Support of a Water-Smart Society The Future of Human Capital in Support of a Water-Smart Society Working Group Human Capital, Water Europe.*

Yang, Andrew. 2020. *The War on Normal People.* Bot uitgevers.

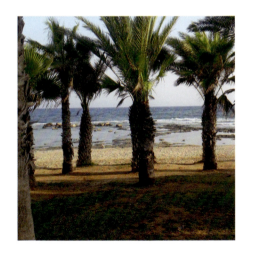
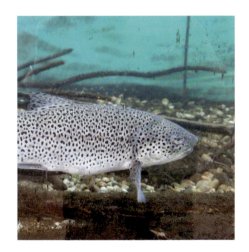
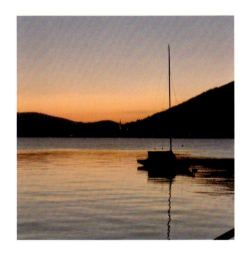
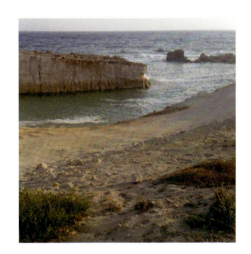
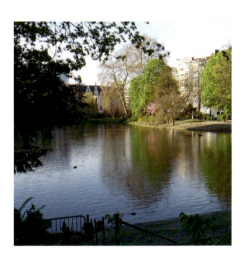
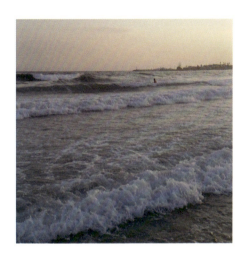

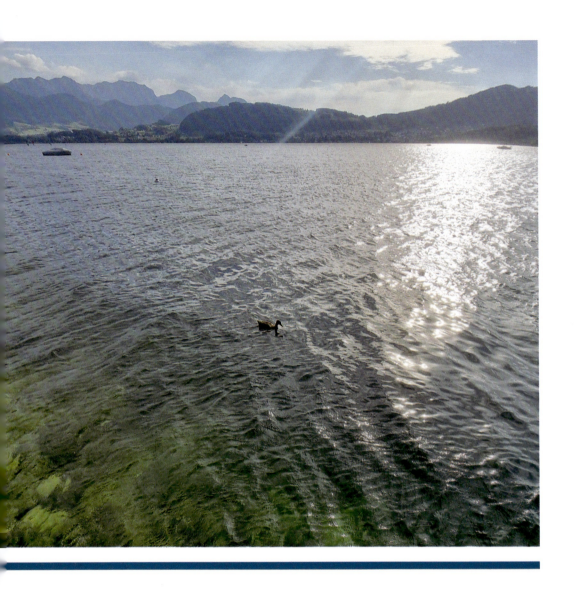

BLUE DEAL ECONOMY — ANALYTICS OF EUROPEAN SOCIAL GOVERNANCE IMPACT ON WATER BUSINESS

Björn Holste (Founder and Managing Partner at Technology Institute),
Stephan Horvath (Founder of Ideations and Board Advisor)

The European "Green Deal" was the waving banner for fighting climate change in the European Union and also a blueprint for the definition of "good" investments and the "taxation" of air components, despite some controversial discussions by EU politicians about the classification of gas and nuclear energy.

The carbon footprint, along with other factors, plays a major role in rating ESG-compliant investments – a significant step in the right direction.

INTEGRATED MANAGEMENT OF WATER RISKS

Air and water might be the essential resources for life on Earth. Over the timespan of Earth's existence and until very recently, both have been taken for granted and their use has been accessible to everyone. Humanity has since come to understand that our impact on climate change is endangering our existence on this planet and has started to take measures to keep the air clean enough to limit the Greenhouse Gas Effect. This aftermath leads to highly complex causalities, including rising sea levels and the loss of biodiversity. This could deprive us of solutions like a cure for cancer derived from a plant or an animal that soon might become extinct before we can learn from it and have the chance to take a shot at understanding its potential.

While much remains to be learned, the scientific community's interdependencies of climate change and water resources have been well researched. In the latest UN water report, Gilbert Houngbo mentions this relationship in the first sentence.

WHY ARE WATER AND WATER RESILIENCE ESSENTIAL?

In scientific literature, the Tragedy of the Commons problem was initially brought up by Lloyd in the early 19th century and was reintroduced by Hardin in 1968. The concept of the Commons as a placeholder for freely available resources has been the foundation for the efforts to internalise costs from GHG emissions, e.g. to control the emission of GHGs by assigning a cost to them.

It seems logical that after considering the importance of air, in the form of partially internalising the cost of air pollution to tame GHG emissions, the focus of general political discussions is now expanding to other lethal risks to humanity like water.

The availability and quality of water have been a prominent topic for decades. Theoretical concepts developed to gain control over GHG emissions, like controlling the total amount issued through allowance certificates while at the same time promoting measures to counterbalance the GHG emissions, might also be applicable to protect an essential resource on this planet: water.

Water use has increased six-fold over the last 100 years and grows at a rate of about 1% annually. Around 771 million people worldwide still lack access to safe water, and an estimated 282 million of them – usual females – travel significant distances to obtain water from a well.

The availability of infrastructure to obtain water, recycle and clean it weighs considerably as a factor in the equation of its impact on climate change and the quality of life. 1.7 billion people – nearly one fourth of the global population – lack a toilet, causing 494 million individuals to defecate out in the open. As human waste releases methane, the warming effect is at least 28 times greater than CO_2, accelerating the global warming cycle. Large amounts of methane are also released when permafrost thaws.

However, this underlines the circular causalities of humankind on the planet, even when the everyday problems faced by people living in developing countries and industrialised nations differ immensely. We are all connected and cannot afford to think as separate nations.

WATER IS THE NEXT ECONOMIC FRONTIER

Water is the "next economic frontier" as it holds potential for wealth, economic growth, employment, and innovation. *(See Chart 1: Limited Quantity of Water Available on the Earth)*

Achieving universal and equitable access to safe and affordable drinking water for all is an essential milestone of the UN SDG goal by 2030. This is to be achieved by substantially increasing water-use efficiency across all sectors and ensuring the sustainable withdrawal and supply of freshwater to address water scarcity and to substantially reduce the number of people suffering from water scarcity.

At the 2022 United Nations Ocean Conference, a "Blue Deal" was promoted to enable to sustainable use of ocean resources for economic growth.
By introducing the words "Blue Deal" this year as an equivalent sibling to the Green Deal, combining this with global trade, investment, and innovation to create a sustainable and resilient water economy is a move toward a more sustainable water economy.

We learned a lot from the Green Deal, and we have the opportunity to avoid some of the mistakes made during the Green Deal process when we are considering a "Blue Deal Economy," a global trade, investment, and innovation movement with a water footprint as the sibling of the carbon footprint will gain political support and traction in Europe.

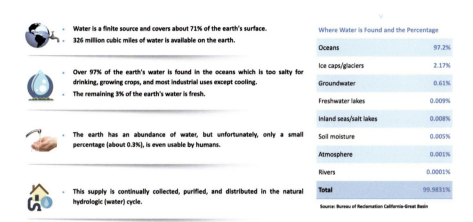

Where Water is Found and the Percentage	
Oceans	97.2%
Ice caps/glaciers	2.17%
Groundwater	0.61%
Freshwater lakes	0.009%
Inland seas/salt lakes	0.008%
Soil moisture	0.005%
Atmosphere	0.001%
Rivers	0.0001%
Total	**99.9831%**

- Water is a finite source and covers about 71% of the earth's surface.
- 326 million cubic miles of water is available on the earth.

- Over 97% of the earth's water is found in the oceans which is too salty for drinking, growing crops, and most industrial uses except cooling.
- The remaining 3% of the earth's water is fresh.

- The earth has an abundance of water, but unfortunately, only a small percentage (about 0.3%), is even usable by humans.

- This supply is continually collected, purified, and distributed in the natural hydrologic (water) cycle.

Source: Bureau of Reclamation California-Great Basin

Chart 1: Limited Quantity of Water Available on the Earth

The following thoughts reflect only the drinking water situation globally and with a particular focus on Europe.

THE GLOBAL DRINKING WATER SCENARIO

Growing pollution and decreasing groundwater replenishment rates have reduced drinking water availability in the past few years. Such a scenario associated with an increasing population is presumed to result in a massive demand/supply mismatch of potable or usable water.
Furthermore, water stress is prominent in China, India, the Middle East and North Africa, and Australia.

Currently, 844 million people, about one in nine of the planet's population, lack access to clean, affordable water within a 30 minute radius around their homes.
Clean and safe drinking water is considered an easy way to remain hydrated and helps to maintain good health. Moreover, the growing incidence of healthcare issues and diseases worldwide is a significant concern.

Access to freshwater resources is vital for the future of entire counties, the people, the food supply, and the production processes. In 2020 the global drinking water market was valued to be around 181 billion Euro. The global market is estimated to grow from 200 billion Euros in 2021 to 421 billion Euros in 2028, growing at a CAGR of 11.2% within the forecasted period (2021-28).

Globally, the total annual consumption of bottled water stood at about 200 billion litres of water. The Asia Pacific region, including India and China, dominates the market, supported by the large population, growing demand, untapped market, and rapid urbanisation.

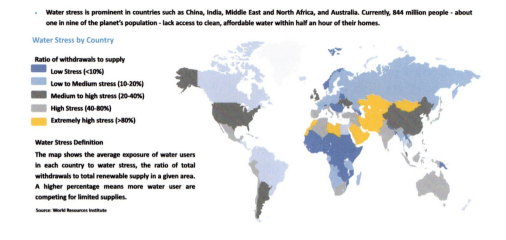

Chart 2: Water Sources are Limited Across the Globe (Quality of Water Across Different Regions of the World Including Europe and within Europe)

WATER MARKET SCENARIO BY MAJOR REGIONS

Western Europe Contributes the Major Share of the Bottled Water Market in Europe. *(See Chart 3)*
The continent enjoys the highest per capita consumption of bottled water globally, with a total annual consumption of more than 50 billion litres. Regarding consumption, Europe alone accounts for more than one-quarter of the global market. Western Europe ranks as the world's most mature bottled water region, driven by significant markets such as Germany, Italy, France, and Spain.

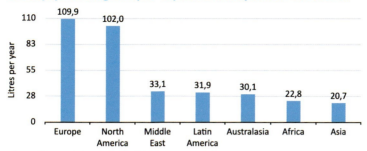

EU Enjoys the Highest per Capita Consumption in the World

Source: European Federation of Bottled Waters

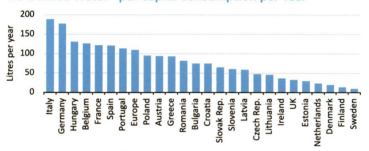

EU Bottled Water - per Capita Consumption per Year

Source: European Federation of Bottled Waters

Chart 3: Western Europe Contributes the Major Share of the Bottled Water Market in Europe

ASIAN DEMAND FOR DRINKING WATER

China is the largest Asian market for bottled water, with about 50 billion litres total of annual consumption in 2020. The little public confidence in drinking water quality, rapid urbanisation, growing disposable income, and the adoption of healthy lifestyles are guiding Chinese preferences towards the consumption of premium water and foreign brands. *(See Chart 4)*

China and Thailand is the Asian countries with largest consumption of bottled water.

Top Bottled Water Consuming Countries

Country	Consumption in million gallons		CAGR
	2015	2020	2015/20
China	20,506.40	27,780.40	6.30%
USA	11,523.60	14,957.80	5.40%
Mexico	8,081.20	9,959.00	4.30%
Indonesia	6,815.60	8,514.10	4.60%
Brazil	5,357.40	6,456.00	3.80%
India	4,596.30	6,416.10	6.90%
Thailand	3,624.00	3,959.30	1.80%
Italy	3,302.20	3,475.00	1.00%
Germany	2,970.20	2,747.40	-1.50%
France	2,079.80	2,238.10	1.50%
Top 10 Subtotal	68,856.60	86,503.10	4.70%
All others	19,419.90	21,789.80	2.30%
World	88,276.50	108,292.90	4.20%

Several Asian Countries like China and India are leading consumer of bottled water, which makes a good business and trade proposition for Thailand.

Per Capita Consumption by Leading Countries

2020 Rank	Countries	Gallons Per Capita	
		2015	2020
1	Mexico	64.2	74.4
2	Italy	55.5	58.8
3	Thailand	52.8	57
4	USA	35.9	45.2
5	UAE	31	35.4
1	Mexico	64.2	74.4

Thailand consumes an average of 57 gallons of water per capita per year, which makes Thailand the third largest per-person consumer of bottled water in the world.

Chart 4: China and Thailand are the Asian countries with largest consumption of bottled water.

In the future, the market in Asia-Pacific will likely maintain its dominance in the global market in terms of market share, supported by increasing demand for bottled water from India, China, Thailand, and Indonesia. The market is driven by growing consumption, increasing consumer awareness, the increasing popularity of premium products, and rising disposable income.

DRINKING WATER DEMAND IN THE GCC

Sweltering, dry climatic conditions and the limited availability of water resources in the GCC have fuelled the demand for bottled water in the region.

The bottled water market is also driven by the growing demand for potable water from the rapid increase in the number of tourists, pilgrims, and expatriate communities in the region, especially in the UAE and Saudi Arabia. *(See Chart 5: Limited Availability of Water Resources in the GCC.)*

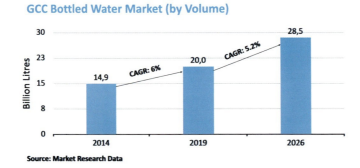

GCC Bottled Water Market (by Volume)

Source: Market Research Data

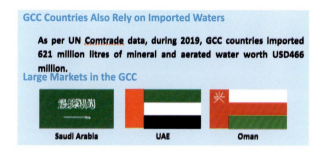

Chart 5: Limited Availability of Water Resources in the GCC. Reliance on Bottled Water Has Increased Due to the Extremely Hot and Dry Climatic Conditions.

The premium bottled water market demand in the GCC is being aided by the rising health consciousness among the consumers, mainly due to the region's high incidences of obesity and diabetes. Consumers have started looking for healthier and more convenient alternatives to sugar-heavy carbonated drinks, providing further impetus to the bottled water market.

DEMAND FOR DRINKING WATER IN THE INDIAN MARKET

Over the past decade, rapid urbanisation increased awareness about the importance of safe drinking water and an increasing per capita income has spurred the demand for bottled water in India. Moreover, India's economy is shifting towards a robust middle class, giving rise to more premium, ethical, personalised products. Furthermore, the concerns over the quality of tap or municipal water also contribute significantly to the country's exponential growth of bottled water.

Most tourists and expatriates are concerned about India's water quality and prefer to use premium quality water brands during their stay.

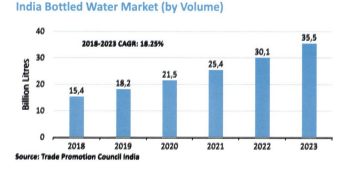

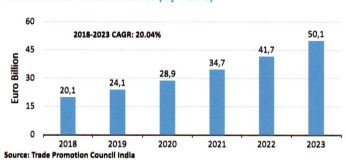

India Bottled Water Market (by Value)

Chart 6: Rapid Urbanisation and Growing Importance of Safe Drinking Water has fueled the Bottled Water Market Growth in India.

The key players catering to the global bottled water market are Nestlé, Coca-Cola, Pepsico, Danone, Mountain Valley Spring Water, Bisleri International, Nongfu Spring, Tata Global Beverages, Mineralquellen und Getränke GmbH & Co. KG, Gerolsteiner Brunnen GmbH & Co. KG, and RHODIUS.

To no small extent, Western Europe is ranked as the world's most mature bottled water region, driven by significant markets such as Germany, Italy, France, and Spain. Regarding consumption, Europe alone accounts for more than one quarter of the global market. The European bottled water market is fragmented and highly competitive, with local and international players. Different countries are captured by different players, with a significant presence of local players in respective countries.
Besides the prominent global players, the other notable players include Hoevelmann, Gerolsteiner Brunnen, Ferrarelle, Acqua Sant'Anna, San Benedetto, Spadel, and Roxane S.A., CoGeDi International.

Of course, there are risks: a growing pollution and decreasing groundwater replenishment rates have reduced drinking water availability in Europe over the past few years. Such a scenario associated with an increasing population is presumed to result in a massive demand/supply mismatch of potable or usable water.

So how can we mitigate the risks by investing in drinking water companies, for example, to prevent groundwater from being overused in the future in entire regions running dry because we wasted the water and have not used it sustainably?

Present environmental, sustainable, and profitable investment opportunities have to follow critical government decisions for sustainable production, water rights, and the

UN SDGs and must include a component that contributes a share of the profit back to society.

The "Blue Deal Economy" for drinking water has to consider the water footprint for the complete value chain, from ownership of water resources to delivering it to the end consumer. This can create new jobs and revenue for European countries.

WATER RISKS ARE REAL - LET US BE PROVOCATIVE

Shouldn't we say that water belongs to everyone as a common, free resource and just the infrastructure cost should be used for pricing water, or less provocative: We all should think about how we can produce and consume water more sustainably and protect our environment.

WATER AND ESG - HOW TO CALCULATE THE RISK

The problem is that environmental water risk for companies is poorly understood and highly complex. A view on both ESG data and business models together is needed as well as analytics along the entire value chain.

We have to estimate how much damage the unmonitored water extraction can be do to the financial system on an aggregated level and to each company attached to the water supply system.

A transitional water risk weighted by a price, like the CO_2 price, will help but leaves out physical climate risks.

So, in short, it is a significant economic factor for which banks, corporations, and re-gulations need analytical help to understand these risks. The knowledge of climate risk will soon become a requirement for every company in the supply chain.

WHAT DO WE NEED TO GET STARTED?

Assessments of risk come in different flavors. Usually, the qualitative approach is applied when specific data is not available. Take an example from the world of physical climate risks: Imagine assessing the risk profile of a nuclear power plant that was built next to a river. Our climate simulations show a high probability of drought in the area over the next 10 years, which is bad news for the adjacent farmers and good news for the people concerned with flood risk (including the electrical engineers at the plant). However, the nuclear plant relies on complex cooling mechanisms which in turn rely on the water from the nearby river. On the other hand, too much water in the form of riverine floods would not be helpful as well, since we then have to assess the flood protection measures for the cooling water pumps.

This example does not even talk about the water quality which must be a great concern when our thought process circles back to the availability of clean drinking water.

If we leave the physical risks – in terms of amounts of water available – aside for now and look at the water quality, the discussion quickly circles back to the available infrastructure.

In an example recently given to me be a fellow technologist, we look at sewage water plants. These collect water to filter, clean, and recycle into the drinking water infrastructure. The level of engineering combines mechanical, biological, and physical principles and can reliably clean sewage water. However, it relies on adding the right ingredients at the right time. A process which is most efficiently handled through a digital infrastructure to measure and control the foul-smelling technical wonderworld. In this example, we learn that most of the sewage plants in the unnamed country, in which our example is set, have turned off all electronics, because they are constantly being hacked (from unfriendly people in another country to remain unnamed here). The manual operation of the plants is more costly and less efficient, leading not only to societal economic impacts but also to lower quality of the end product – water.

So, who would have thought that cybersecurity is an important factor when assessing water quality? Even when technical equipment to collect data and control processes is available, it must be secure. Consequences of releasing polluted water to the public could seriously impact health, and their economic implications on global supply chains could be witnessed, for example, by the lack of lorry drivers in the UK during the Corona pandemic.

AVAILABLE DATA

After considering some of the challenges in the qualitative assessment of risks associated with water availability and quality, let's move on to the next step that is required to actually make some calculations: quantitative data.

On a global scale and especially in the developed countries, the local statistical offices are doing a good job of collecting all sorts of data from companies, authorities, and individuals. They represent a powerful infrastructure for obtaining data and are paid for with your tax money. Unfortunately, their output is not usable directly as formats differ across countries. Some efforts to clean the data have been made on the European level and with standardisation organisations internationally. But the much-coveted job of data scientist still consists of more than 80% in cleaning data and making it useable in a calculation.

The collection of data requires in turn the availability of data points. These should come not only from official sources but also from the companies themselves. For the collection of metrics, an immutable database solution (blockchain) would be advisable so that companies can stay in control of their data and grant different levels of access to authorities and the general public. Availability of Big Data, provided through publicly accessible blockchain databases with controlled access would also lay the ground for the application of machine learning and AI techniques, allowing us to paint a more global and connected picture of the water landscape. Better and bigger data would also be a sound starting point for future simulations under existing scenarios, tying together the different health, socioeconomic, and climate impacts of water availability and quality.

Unfortunately, the availability of reliable data points not only for water quality – or the lack thereof in terms of pollution and hazardous and non-hazardous waste – is only one of the prerequisites towards the internalisation of cost in a way similar to the certificates allowing GHG emissions.

The second important ingredient is the cost of restoring the water to an acceptable quality. This might happen on different scales for seawater and freshwater and takes into account various downstream effects like the loss of biodiversity and health impacts on society.

To arrive at plausible and quantified risk assessments, we then must combine the data with forward looking simulations. The collections of models and scenarios by the NGFS is usually a good starting point for this.

SCOPE FOR WATER

For the assessment of GHG emissions, and the major frameworks like the TCFD and the EU Taxonomy, interestingly the focus of splitting inward and outwards effects into three scopes is reserved for GHG emissions. It seems only a matter of time until this approach is extended to other risk factors. In the scientific community, the algorithms for combining global trade information in the form of input-output tables with factors other than CO_2 and GHG emissions are well known. They could be applied for a variety of factors, some of them – like water pollution and waste – could have a more immediate effect in providing the grounds to support the internalisation of costs along global supply chains.

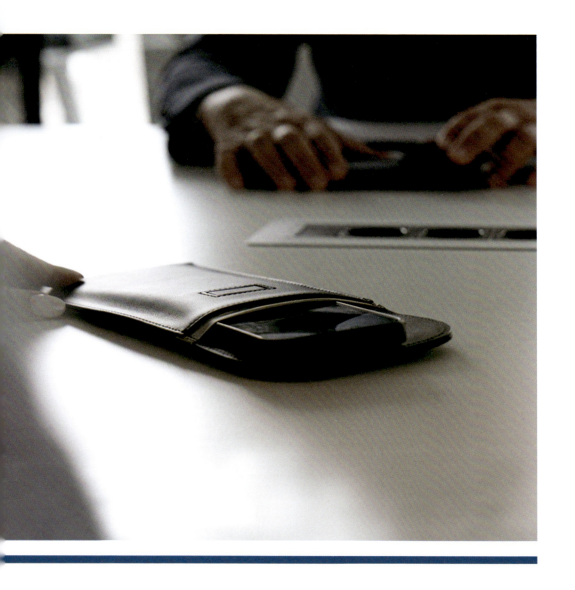

PURE PRIVACY PROTECTION #NOHACKING #NOTRACKING

Lisa Strassl

Be prepared...
...to protect your privacy against your personal cyber emergency!

Cyber risk has been dynamically increasing in recent years with the ongoing trend of digitalisation. Whether in private life or in the business context, it becomes more and more important to individually defend against all upcoming threats.

Did you know, for example, that even if you switch off your smartphone, you still can be trackable? Or if your device is already infected by malware that runs in the background, flight mode would be ineffective to prevent you from malevolent hackers?

THE INNOVATIVE SOLUTION MADE IN EUROPE

Privacy bags (for example by ALLPURE) are your guarantee for more privacy and security and contribute to your health. In detail, they:
- protect from hacking, tracking, and remote access to your device
- block various electromagnetic & wireless signals like 5G, WIFI, UMTS, Bluetooth, GPS, RFID;
- reduce viruses and bacteria on the surface of your device once you put it in the bag – thanks to the zinc, silver and copper coating of the tissue
- are suitable for all standard device sizes

Prof Dipl.-Ing Peter Pauli, Professor for High Frequency – Microwave- and Xray Technology at the Bundeswehr University Munich, Germany, puts it all in a nutshell:

"Innovative protection bags, as for example Privacy bags by ALLPURE, are the perfect solution for more privacy in day to day life. As soon as your device is stored in it, it blocks as a Faraday cage all your incoming and outgoing signals."

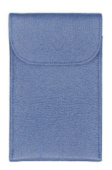
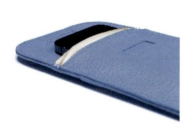
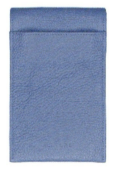

AUTHORS

Author	Short Biography
Lars Skov Andersen 	China Resources Management Senior consultant with +25 years experience in managing international water resources and integrated rural development projects at national, local and river basin levels on behalf of World Bank, DfiD, EU and Danida. Chief Technical Adviser to water and environment ministries of Vietnam, China, Zambia and Denmark. Currently coordinating the China Europe Water Platform policy dialogue on groundwater as part of the Rural Water and Food Security Project supported by the EU Partnership Instrument.
Mona Arnold 	VTT Technical Research Centre of Finland Mona Arnold (Lic. Tech., MBA) has her expertise in circular economy processes and technologies and interest in developing circular and sustainable business models and value chains. She acts as a principal scientist at VTT Technical Research Centre of Finland. She has a wide experience in the valorisation of different waste material and end of life products, such as municipal sludge and end of life vehicles. Lately she has been involved in several projects relating to the management of plastic waste and waste prevention and she is, among others leading a project on solutions for floating plastic debris, and analysing the formation of plastic waste valorisation innovation ecosystems. She is also involved in water management and its digitalization and active member of the European technology platform Water Europe.
Ruud P. Bartholomeus 	Chief Science Officer of KWR, Principal Scientist of the Ecohydrology team and Senior Coordinating Researcher at Wageningen University Aligning regional freshwater supply and demand is central to his work. This involves combining scientific knowledge and technological solutions such as (cross-sectoral) water reuse, sub-irrigation with (industrial) residual water, and online management of climate-adaptive drainage with the process of having water managers, drinking water utilities, industry, and farmers work together to achieve sufficient freshwater.
Malgorzata Anna Bogusz (Co-Author) 	President, The Kulski Foundation for Polish – American Relations Małgorzata Bogusz has been affiliated with the Kulski Foundation since 2017, initially as Advisor to the Foundation's Board, and later as President of the Board appointed in December 2018 by the Foundation Council. She has implemented a number of projects aimed at promoting patriotic values and attitudes, both in Poland and abroad.

Author	Short Biography
Ines Breda	IWA Emerging Water Leaders Steering Committee Member Inês works as a Product and Process Manager at Silhorko-EUROWATER A/S – A Grundfos Company. PhD, strong knowledge on filtration technology for production of drinking water. Passionate about data science and international collaborations. Board member and Treasurer of the IWA Young Water Professionals in Denmark. Board Member of IWA SG Design Operation and Management of Drinking Water Treatment Plants.
Marianna Brichese	Scientific Communication Expert Marianna Brichese is graduated in Industrial Chemistry at University of Padova and received a master's degree in "Surface treatments for industry". After 12 years of experience in R&D for a multinational company as researcher and project manager, and after international work experience, she is finalized a master's degree in Science Communication with the target to put together technical background with writing abilities. Her higher interest is on environment, sustainability and technological topics.
Véronique Briquet-Laugier	ANR Véronique Briquet-Laugier was educated in both France and the USA. With a PhD in Biophysics, she worked for 17 years to elucidate cardiovascular diseases and rare haemorrhagic disorders. She has also been a consultant for technology transfer in the field of biotechnologies. Véronique was at the creation of the French funding agency (ANR) where she developed a portfolio of national, European and international programs for the Health Department. As a French diplomat, she spent four years in India (2010-2014) as the Science & Technology Counsellor of the French Ambassador, where she launched the Indo-French Water Network, a first experience in the field of Water management and policy. Recently, she also spent two years as a diplomat in South Africa as the Cultural, Science & Innovation Counsellor of the French Ambassador in Pretoria. Expert for the French government (Nanomedicine & Forensics) Véronique still sits on evaluation panels for the European Commission in Brussels. She joined the Water JPI in October 2020.

Author	Short Biography
Paul Campling (Co-Author)	VITO

| **Cristian Carboni**
 | Light Industries Market Manager of Industrie De Nora S.p.a.

More than 20 years of experience in project management, research, and technological innovation, author of numerous scientific publications. In Industrie De Nora he collaborates in the development of technologies relating to water and wastewater treatment, in particular concerning disinfection.
Member of the scientific committee of Polo Agrifood, member of the Board of Directors of the International Ozone Association, Leader of the Water Europe Working Group Water and Public Health.
Since 2017 he has collaborated with the Executive Agency for Small and Medium-sized Enterprises (EASME) for the monitoring of the Actions under Horizon 2020; currently external expert of the European Innovation Council and Executive Agency for SMEs (EISMEA). |

| **Gaetano Casale**
 | IHE Delft Institute for Water Education

Gaetano Casale has been working at IHE Delft since May 2007. Together with his colleagues in the Liaison Officer, he provides assistance and advice to academic staff in project acquisition, formulation and implementation. He facilitates clients requesting for services and liaises with partner institutes and donors interested in cooperating with IHE Delft.
Gaetano is an expert in Project Cycle Management and has a broad knowledge of donor programmes. Recently he has also started representing IHE Delft in relevant water sector platforms at European level.
He is directly responsible for a broad range of key corporate functions: Business Development, Project Management, Contract Management, Partnership Management, Quality Management, Personal Data Protection.
Gaetano has an MSc in Electrical Engineering and an MSc in Water Services Management. Previously he has worked as Quality Manager in the commercial sector. He has also been board member of a small NGO conducting water and sanitation projects in developing countries. |

| **Rafael Casielles Restoy**
 | Chemical Engineer and Senior project manager at BIOAZUL

More than 14 years of experience in R&I projects devoted to different fields like water treatment, sustainable sanitation, solid waste management, and agriculture. In the few last years, Rafael Casielles Restoy has focused on water reuse in agriculture analysing the technology needs for water reclamation and the barriers for upscaling innovations. He has coordinated several R&I projects on circular economy applied to the agricultural sector such as SUWANU EUROPE, RICHWATER, and TREAT&USE. |

Author	Short Biography
	He was a member of Body of Knowledge of EIT programme on water scarcity in 2021. He is currently co-leading an international consortium called BONEX to develop practical tools to implement the WEFE Nexus approach in the Mediterranean.
Diana Chavarro Rincon (Co-Author)	ITC Enschede
Jordi Cros	Telecommunications Engineer, with more than 35 years of experience in design and development of HW and SW of electronic equipment, communications systems, and control systems, of which more than 25 years in the field of water and environment. Coordinator and participant in projects of the international programs FP4, FP5, FP7, H2020, LIFE or CIP_Eco-Innovation, projects in the national programs of CDTI CENIT or regional as FEDER-Innterconecta or RIS3CAT. Author of several patents related to automatic water quality measurement systems. Currently Portfolio Development Manager of the Water Sensors Area and Head of Innovation at ADASA Sistemas, President of the Catalan Water Partnership, co-leader of the Water Sensors and Tools Working Group of Water Europe, and facilitator of the GT4 ICT and Smart Technologies group of the Spanish Water Technology Platform.
Dominique Darmendrail	Waters and Global Changes Scientific Programme Director at BRGM Experienced Scientific Advisor with a demonstrated history of working in the environmental services. Skilled in Environmental Issues, Water Quantity and Quality management, risk management and Sustainable development. Strong research professional with European and International focus. Co-director of the OneWater Exploratory research programme (Recovery Plan France 2030). Head of Innovation at ADASA, President of the Catalan Water parnership.
Sacha de Rijk	Head of Department of Freshwater Ecology and Water Quality at Deltares Experienced advisor and research coordinator with a demonstrated history of working in the research industry. Skilled in Natural Resource Management, Aquatic Ecology, Sustainable Development, Management, and Water Quality. Strong education professional with a PhD focused in Earth Sciences from Vrije Universiteit Amsterdam.

Author	Short Biography
Roberto Di Bernardo	Senior Researcher and Head of the R&D Open Government Unit, part of Open Public Service Innovation Lab He is an electronic engineer with Professional Master's degrees in "Clinical Engineering" and in "Internet Software Engineering." He has been working as a researcher at Engineering R&D Laboratory since 2004, has been involved in management and technical activities in many Italian and European projects. He is also acts as R&D opportunities and network developer for the entire Open Public Service Innovation Lab. The lab is involved, among others, in the following projects: PathoCERT (H2020-SU-DRS02), WQeMS (H2020- LC-SPACE-18-EO), B-WaterSmart (H2020-CE-SC5-04), Gotham (PRIMA). At the moment, Roberto is coordinating URBANAGE project (H2020-DTTransforations-02), leading the Smart Governance and Smart Cities sub-group of the Big Data Value Association, co-leading the Smart Cities Domain Committee of the FIWARE Foundation and the Digital Water Systems Working Group of Water Europe.
Anna Di Mauro	Project Engineer at Med.Hydro s.r.l. Anna Di Mauro is an Environmental Engineer with specialization in Hydrology, Hydraulics, Maritime and Debris Flow. Shareholder and Project Engineer at Med.Hydro s.r.l.. Responsible of the Water Europe Working Group Water sensors and tools (WATERSET) Secretariat. PhD Industry 4.0 PhD – National European Operative Project PON 2014-2020: Innovative models, technologies and methodologies for the analysis and management of Hydraulic Big Data (HBD) to be integrated into Water Utilities as Decision Support System. Expert in numerical hydraulic model: water resources management, water utilities, rivers and reservoirs, water resources and land use management, water distribution piping systems, water supply network partitioning, coastal and marine infrastructure. Main research themes: - smart water networks methods for water supply network partitioning, - analysis of hydraulic big data for profiling user's behaviours, - pressure management for water pressure optimisation in order to reduce leakage in destruct meter areas (DMAs), - demand side management for Water Utilities, - innovative techniques to detect leakage in smart water networks, - numerical and physical models for the study of the coasts, - bidimensional flood simulation model to define hydraulic risk from debris flow in natural basin and artificial channel.

Author	Short Biography
Armando Di Nardo	Professor in Water Resources Management Armando Di Nardo, PhD and Professor in Water Resources Management. Coauthor of more than 200 publications on national and international Journals with research work on optimal management and protection of water resources; optimal partitioning of water supply network; optimal management of water reservoir; optimal design of permeable reactive barrier. Member and Cofounder of some spinoff companies and Leader of the Working Group "Water Sensors and Tools WG Leader" of Water Europe.
Michael Dickstein	Sustainability/ESG Lead | Public Affairs and Communication Expert During 20 years mainly in the FMCG sector, Michael Dickstein has gained broad experience in reputation and stakeholder strategy, ESG, corporate affairs, and communication. Among other roles, he was Heineken's Global Director Sustainable Development and Group Director Sustainability & Community for CocaCola HBC. His focus areas comprise of climate action, water stewardship, circular packaging schemes, and community engagement but also crisis management and corporate advocacy. Michael graduated from law school in Linz/Austria. He started his career in the European Parliament.
Milou M.L. Dingemans	Chief Science Officer of KWR and guest researcher at the Institute for Risk Assessment Sciences at Utrecht University Dr. Dingemans is a European Registered Toxicologist and has over 15 years of experience in scientific research into the harmful effects of chemicals on health. She works on the evaluation of possible health and water quality issues of substances in the water cycle on commissions from water utilities, government, and industry, and the development, validation, and implementation of innovative monitoring and risk assessment methodologies.
Sara Eeman	Programme Manager Resilient Water Systems at Aveco de Bondt/Dareiu Sara has worked in water-related research, education, and business for more than 15 years. After the MSc Applied Earth Science at TU Delft she finished a PhD on groundwater salinity at Wageningen UR. She added to the development of the Land- and Water Management Course at Van Hall Larenstein Applied University as teacher and coordinator. Also she was involved in several research programmes concerning sustainable river management, and was one of the founders of the joint venture master programme River Delta Development (VHL, RH and HZ Applied Universities).

Author	Short Biography
	For two years she has been the programme manager Resilient Water Systems at Aveco de Bondt/ Dareius, focusing on integral approaches for water management, including the development of biodiversity/ecology structures within the company. Since this year, she has led the new workgroup on Water and Biodiversity.
Richard Elelman 	EURECAT Richard Elelman joined CTM as Head of Public Administrations in 2011. CTM has now become part of EURECAT, the Technology Centre of Catalonia. He now serves as Head of Politics and as such continues to work creating bridges between the world of Research and Development and political institutions such as the European Union, (by whom he is employed as an External Expert) the UN, the OECD, the UFM and both national and regional governments. He has recently specialized in the politics of Climate Change, Energy and Water and the effects on Migration, citizen engagement in Europe and the Middle East, and the WATER-ENERGY-FOOD-ECOSYSTEMS Nexus. He has been the Director General of NETWERC H2O and has served on the Board of Directors of WATER EUROPE as well as the EIP WATER Steering Group, appointed by Commissioner Vella of the European Union. Richard is now leading the Social Engagement Programme of The World Water Quality Alliance under the umbrella of the United Nations and preparing programmes regarding Climate Change, Migration, and Gender Equality.
Jan Willem Foppen 	IHE Delft Jan Willem Foppen (1965) received his M.Sc. degree in Hydrogeology from the VU University in Amsterdam in 1990. After his graduation, he started to work at Natuurmonumenten (nature conservation organization), and then as a consultant at the Institute of Applied Geosciences of TNO. In 1995-1996, he was stationed in Sana'a, Yemen, where he was part of a project team aimed to identify sources for the drinking water supply of Sana'a. He worked for Natuurmonumenten, Dienst Grondwaterverkenning TNO, the Institute of Applied Geosciences of TNO, and since 1998 for IHE Delft. Intrigued by poor groundwater health conditions in various developing countries, Foppen focused on the transport of the fecal indicator organism Escherichia coli in saturated porous media. Over the years, his interest focused more on the transport of colloids in groundwater and surface waters. Besides the transport of bacteria and silica DNA tracers, his research interests include water and sanitation in slums in Sub-Saharan Africa.

Author	Short Biography
Rafael Gimenez-Esteban	Head of the Digital Team at CETaqua

Rafael Gimenez is the Head of the Digital Team at Cetaqua, the Water Technology Centre, which works in the application of Artificial Intelligence and scalable technologies to the water cycle and sustainability.
As a software engineer and Senior Researcher, he's been working for more than 8 years as a R&D Team Manager in the field of AI.
Before joining Cetaqua, Rafael served for more than 8 years as Researcher and Research Area Manager at BDigital Technology Centre, with a special contribution to the definition and launch of the Big Data Center of Excellence. |
| **Panagiotis Gkofas** (Co-Author) | Member of the European Economic and Social Committee

Economist, MBA, member of the board of directors of the Hellenic Confederation of Professionals, Craftsmen and Merchants (GSEVEE) for SMEs; member of the board of directors of the Panhellenic Confederation of Restaurants and Related Businesses (POESE); representative of the GSEVEE at UEAPME for SMEs; president of the Brussels-based Avignon Academy for SMEs; president of the EU-Turkey JCC; European Commission expert on food loss and waste. |
| **Sanja Gottstein** | University of Zagreb, Croatia

Prof. Dr. Sc. Sanja Gottstein currently works at the Department of Biology, Faculty of Science, University of Zagreb. Dr Gottstein does research in Ecology, Zoology and Systematics (Taxonomy) of Crustacea. |
| **Rasha Hassan** | Project officer at H2O-People; PhD candidate at the University of Barcelona

Rasha is an accomplished Project Officer at H2OPeople with expertise in water resource management through her involvement in several Erasmus+ and Horizon Europe projects. Her primary responsibilities include conducting research, managing the administrative and financial aspects of H2OPeople projects, and ensuring smooth day-to-day operations. Rasha is also involved in communication and dissemination activities, public events and networking. Rasha is committed to bridging the gap between science, policy, and practices in water and food securities and has a proven track record of implementing climate adaptation strategies in the MENA region.

Rasha holds a Bachelor's degree in Civil Engineering and a Master's degree in Environmental Systems Engineering from Tishreen University, Syria, and a Master's degree in Water and Coastal Management from the University of Bologna, Italy. |

Author	Short Biography
	She is currently pursuing a PhD in Geography, Territorial Planning, and Environmental Management from the Faculty of Geography and History at the University of Barcelona, Spain, which is further enhancing her research skills and knowledge in the field of water resource management..
Björn Holste	Founder and Managing Partner at Technology Institute Björn is founder of the Technology Institute and co-founder and Managing Partner of Liminalytics, an organisation specialised in sustainability risk assessment. He was educated at University of Kaiserslautern as an engineer, as well as at Wake Forest University and Harvard Business School. He received his PhD in macroeconomics from the University of Kaiserslautern and teaches at the Frankfurt School of Finance.
Stephan Horvath	Founder of Ideations and Board Advisor Stephan has over 20 years of international C-level experience in working for network agencies and consulting firms. He is the founder of Ideations, an Investor Relations marketing firm advising tech clients and tech funds on business and innovation strategies. Previously Stephan worked as CEO of IPG Digital and Media Services, building relationships with international clients and corporations. He holds a Master's degree in economics and computer science from the Technical University of Stuttgart, Germany, and is a frequent keynote speaker at international conferences.
Achim Kaspar	Member of the Board of VERBUND AG Achim Kaspar is a Member of the Board of VERBUND AG – Austria's leading electricity company and one of the largest producers of electricity from hydropower in Europe. He assumed the role as COO in January 2019 and is responsible for digitisation as well as the VERBUND generation portfolio which includes the oversight of 130 hydropower plants. Prior to joining VERBUND, he held various management positions in the Utility and Service Provider Industry as well as in the Austrian Telecommunication Industry. From 2008 – 2018 Achim Kaspar was the General Manager at Cisco Austria / Slovenia / Croatia.

Author	Short Biography
Juergen F. Kolb	Professor for Bioelectrics at Leibniz Institute for Plasma Science and Technology (INP Greifswald) Prof. Dr. Juergen Kolb received his PhD (Dr. rer. nat.) in Physics from the Friedrich-Alexander University of Erlangen-Nurenberg in 1999. After his preparation service to teach mathematics and physics at secondary schools, he joined Old Dominion University in Norfolk, Virginia, USA in 2002. He left as tenured Associate Professor in the Department of Electrical and Computer Engineering for a joint appointment of the Leibniz Institute for Plasma Science and Technology and the Institute of Physics of the University of Rostock in 2011. The application of non-thermal plasmas for the disinfection and the decontamination of water is one of his specific research interests as head of the Research Program Agriculture-Bioeconomy-Environment.
Durk Krol	Executive Director of Water Europe Durk Krol is the Executive Director of Water Europe. He has worked in the water sector at the European level for the last 20 years, initially as a Senior Legal Policy Officer for the water department of provincial government of Friesland (NL) and as Deputy Secretary General at EUREAU. During his time at EUREAU he became involved in Water Europe, initially as a board member and since 2011 in his current position. He has also closely been involved in the creation of the MEP Water Group in the European Parliament. Durk is a graduate of law, with an additional Master's degree in Latin American studies and an MBA. He has also completed the Executive Development Programme at Vlerick Business School, an Executive Master in International Association Management at Solvay Brussels School, and the Programme on Negotiation Global Online at Harvard Law School.
Andreas Kunsch	Advisor to the Chief Operation Officer of VERBUND AG Andreas Kunsch is currently the advisor to the Chief Operation Officer of VERBUND AG – Austria's leading electricity company and one of the largest producers of electricity from hydropower in Europe. He has been with VERBUND for over 15 years, including more than 10 years in a variety of positions and areas at VERBUND hydropower. Since the autumn of 2017, he has been the assistant to the member of the management board responsible for generation, digitisation, IT, and sustainability, where he also represents VERBUND in various committees' strategy for Africa.

Author	Short Biography
Peter Latzelsperger 	Managing Director at UNIHA Wasser Technologie GmbH and Lecturer at multiple Universities of Applied Sciences Peter graduated from University of Applied Sciences Upper Austria. After his studies, he joined international business at VAMED AG, within the department of Latin America and the Caribbean. After progressing within the regional organization in Latin America and spending some years living in Latin America, Peter came back to Austria in 2020. In 2021, Peter joined UNIHA Wasser Technologie as Commercial Director. Since 2023, Paul Schausberger and Peter took over as UNIHA´s managing directors.
Piet N.L. Lens 	Professor of New Energy Technologies at National University Ireland, Galway Prof. Dr. Piet Lens is an established professor of New Energy Technologies at National University Ireland, Galway (Ireland). He is also an adjunct professor of Environmental Biotechnology at IHE Delft (the Netherlands) and Tampere University (Finland). Besides innovative research, he is also a leader in education and capacity-building, organising numerous study-days, conferences, summer schools, and short courses. He has (co-)authored over 700 scientific publications and edited eleven book volumes, of which 4 have been translated into Chinese.
Piia Leskinen 	PhD, Principal Lecturer at Turku University of Applied Sciences, Finland Piia Leskinen is a Principal Lecturer at Turku University of Applied Sciences, where she is also part of the Water and Environmental Engineering research group. The group has firm expertise on water protection, the marine environment and wastewater treatment. They have carried out numerous R&D projects related to the protection and monitoring of aquatic environment and aquatic organisms, the monitoring of water quality and the restoration of water bodies.
Antonio Lo Porto (Co-Autor)	CNR IRSA

Author	Short Biography
Antonia María Lorenzo López	Founder and CEO at BIOAZUL Antonia Lorenzo has a Bachelor's of Agricultural Chemistry, is a specialist in Environmental Engineering and Technology, and is currently doing her PhD in the economic evaluation of the use of reclaimed water in agriculture at the University of Córdoba, Spain. Antonia is founder, CEO, and R&D director at BIOAZUL. She has worked for more than 20 years in the management and implementation of more than 60 national and international projects, mainly related to blue infrastructures for the sustainable water management – treatment, water reuse, ecological sanitation, nature-based solutions – as well as circular economy and resources sustainability. She works for the European Commission as an external expert and evaluator in several of its programmes. Since 2018 Antonia has led the working group of Water Europe on Water & Sustainable Agrifood Systems. Antonia is a member of the Spanish Management Committee of the Circular City COST Action and also the president of the Spanish "Nature- based solution Cluster" established in the city of Málaga in 2018. Finally, she is a member of the Governing Council of the Andalusian Knowledge Agency. Antonia is also a mentor for the EIT Food Accelerator Network, the Cajamar Innova Incubator, and has recently been selected as a mentor in the European Commission's "EIC Women Leadership Program."
Nataša Mori	National Institute of Biology, Slovenia Nataša Mori is a freshwater ecosystem researcher at the Department of freshwater and terrestrial ecosystems at National Institute of Biology in Ljubljana with a focus on studies of both groundwater and surface, transitional areas between different ecosystems, and the impact of disturbances. She works at the National Institute of Biology in Ljubljana and has also worked at EAWAG, Switzerland. Her research interests include Ostracods (Crustacea), biodiversity conservation, and ecosystem services issues.
Augustin Perner	CEO at PROBIG GmbH Augustin Perner is the founder of Probig GmbH, a worldwide active company for innovative, energy efficient and sustainable solutions for water and waste-water treatment plants. With more than 25 years of experience in international projects he is an expert for rectangular sedimentation- and flotations-tanks for refineries, petrochemical industry, chemical plants, seawater-desalination plants and municipal drinking- and waste water treatment plants. He is also the co-founder and first vice president of the SGD6 water group for SME.

Author	Short Biography
Johannes Pfaffenhuemer	Managing director of Water of Life GmbH Doctorate in business administration, managing director of Water of Life GmbH, expert for holistic health promotion, vital practice in Vogelparadies am Inn, board member of European Global Water Forum, board member of Quellen des Lebens e.V. (Source of Life) Germany / Munich, board member of Austrian Society for Health Promotion / Vienna
Paul Rübig	fMEP; Member of the Administrative Board of the European Institute for Innovation and Technology; Member of the European Economic and Social Committee Dr. Paul Rübig, born in Wels (Upper Austria), was a member of the European Parliament from 1996 to 2019. He is married and has two children. As president of the HTL Alumni Club Steyr, he has always been engaged in the technical education of young people. In 2019, Paul Rübig was appointed to the Advisory Board of Rübig Holding GmbH. He is also a member of the Governing Board of the EIT (European Institute of Innovation & Technology) and a member of the European Economic and Social Committee. In 2022, Paul Rübig was appointed as the External Advisor to the Board of Directors of Water Europe.
Andrea Rubini	Director of Operations at Water Europe Andrea Rubini is a water resource engineer with more than 35 years of experience in the water sector, in climate change and its related impact on urban, industrial, and rural ecosystems. He has been serving as the Director of Operations at Water Europe, the European Water Technology Platform that was set up by the EC and has been promoting water related RTD and innovation in Europe since September 2016. Andrea has also previously worked as a policy advisor to the EC on Smart and Sustainable Growth for the AfDB, ILO, and UNDP.
Dragan Savic	Chief Science Officer of KWR Dragan Savić is the Chief Executive Officer at KWR Water based in the Netherlands and a professor of Hydroinformatics at the University of Exeter in the UK. Professor Savić is an international expert in smart water systems with over 35 years of experience working in engineering, academia, and research consultancy. His work has resulted in patentable innovation and spinout companies. In addition to innovation and leadership skills, he is known for believing in and practising "bridging science and practice" in the wider water sector and utilities in general.

Author	Short Biography
Paul Schausberger	Managing Director UNIHA Wasser Technologie GmbH Paul graduated from the Vienna University of Technology (Austria) with a PhD in process engineering in 2004. During his studies, the university accepted a research assignment involving the development of a mathematical model for thermal seawater desalination processes (multi-effect, multistage-flash, thermal/ mechanical vapor compression). This was the moment when Paul became fascinated with water and twenty years on, this fascination is as strong as ever. His postdoctoral studies led him to the UNESCO Centre for Membrane Science and Technology at the University of New South Wales (Australia), where he investigated fouling phenomena at ultrafiltration. Paul then returned to Vienna and two years later, he left academia for the EPC business by joining the water technology company VA TECH WABAG. There he continued the development of software for the design of thermal desalination processes and worked as a process engineer in various departments. In 2012, Paul moved on to become the CTO at UNIHA Wasser Technologie, an EPC contractor located in Linz/Austria with a strong emphasis on reverse osmosis technology. In 2023, he and Peter Latzelsperger took over as the UNIHA managing directors.
Josef Schnaitl	Gisaqua GmbH Beside leading major project organisations, an important activity of his has been the advice and support of governmental authorities in their efforts for implementation of their water infrastructure programmes considering all kinds of state-of-the-art technologies (in Waste Water Activated Sludge-, SBR-, MBR-, Moving Bed- and Biofiltration, Thermal versus RO Desalination, etc.). Based on his education as an electrical engineer, a dignified experience in a wide range of aspects "in water" has been gained during his more than 40 years in the industry in relation to the water market.
David Smith	Chair of the International Water Relations (Water Beyond Europe) David Smith is the director of the consulting company, Water, Environment, and Business for Development. He has a Bachelor's degree in Botany and Zoology (2000) and an Honours Degree in Limnology (2001) from the University of Cape Town (RSA). He has a Master's Degree in Water and Environmental Management from Loughborough University (UK) (2015) and is currently a PhD candidate at the Autonomous University of Barcelona in Environmental Science and Technology.

Author	Short Biography
	David has led more than 25 projects on environmental studies across the globe. His expertise in economic and social development is focused on environmental management, integrated water resource management, Green Growth, environmental business models, ecosystem services, stakeholder participation and engagement strategies, climate change adaptation and mitigation, and capacity development.
Davide Storelli	Researcher at Engineering Ingegneria Informatica SPA Davide Storelli is a senior Researcher and has been a member of the Open Public Service Innovation unit of the R&D division at Engineering Ingegneria Informatica since 2012. He was Prince2 Practitioner Level certified in 2019. He graduated in Computer Engineering from the University of Salento in 2006. He coordinates the technical activities of several Italian and European projects related to Smart Cities and Smart Water, with special focus on service innovation, open platforms, and digital transformation. He is the co-author of several publications in international journals and conferences.
Lisa Strassl	Lisa Strassl, LL.M. (38) has a more than 10 years proven track record gathered in major law firms as well as top multinational FMCG companies. With her broad and deep management experience on industry side as well as an Advisory Board Member she decided to found her own company ALLPURE in 2022. With her strong believe in the future need, that everyone must be better prepared for future digital threats, the focus of her company is to regain and secure the digital privacy.
Naomi Timmer	Director of H2O-People Naomi Timmer is the director of H2O-People and its flagship programme, the European Junior Water Programme (EJWP). Naomi has been active for almost 10 years in the water management sector as a programme manager for several personal development programmes in the Dutch water sector. Since 2019, she has been the creator and director of the EJWP to share the knowledge and enthusiasm of a holistic leadership approach within a European context. Naomi has a Master's in political science and a Bachelor's degree in religious studies. She specialised in Religion and Violence, power structures, and public affairs. She always thought she accidentally ended up in the water sector until she heard Kofi Annan at Making Waves (7 September 2017).

Author	Short Biography
Geoff Townsend 	Water-Smart Industry Cluster at Water Europe & Industry fellow at NALCO Water Geoff Townsend has over 30 years' experience in industrial water and energy management with various roles in business development, the optimization of resource-intensive industries and innovation. He is actively engaged in a variety of sustainability initiatives particularly in water stewardship, biodiversity, science-based target setting and the water-energy nexus. Geoff participated in the ISO Standard Committee for Water Footprinting (ISO 14046) and partnered with the World Wildlife Fund (WWF) and the Alliance for Water Stewardship (AWS) to certify Ecolab's Taicang facility in China as the world's first manufacturing facility to meet the AWS standard certification requirements. Since 2017, he has led the Water Smart Industry Cluster for Water Europe. Geoff is currently involved in the development of digital solutions that that helps businesses make informed choices on how to balance productivity and sustainability goals. Dr. Townsend has a BSc in Ecology (UEA) and a PhD in Environmental Chemistry from the University of Cambridge.
Eloisa Vargiu 	CETaqua Water Technology Centre Eloisa Vargiu holds a Ph.D. in Electronic and Computer Engineering by the University of Cagliari (Italy). Currently, she is working at Cetaqua, Water Technology Centre, as a specialist in public funding, collaborating with the research in the field of Water 4.0. She is also the leader of the working group on Water & Digital Systems for Water Europe. In 2002, she obtained the accreditation as an associate professor from Quality Agency of the University system (AQU), Generalitat de Catalunya and, in 2020, the accreditation as an associate professor from the Ministry of Instruction and University in Italy. From 2013 to 2020, she managed the Integrated Care research line at the eHealth R&D Unit, Eurecat Centre Tecnòlogic de Catalunya. From April 2016 to December 2019, she was the technical coordination of the EU project CONNECARE (H2020) which was evaluated as "outstanding" by the EC. From January 2012 to June 2015, she was the technical coordinator of and main researcher for the EU project.

Author	Short Biography
Uta Wehn (Co-Author)	IHE Delft
Klaus-Dieter Weltmann	Chairman of the Board and Scientific Director INP Greifswald Prof. Dr. Klaus-Dieter Weltmann received his doctorate in applied physics from the University of Greifswald in 1993. In the mid-1990s he moved to ABB Schweiz AG (Asea Brown Boveri) in the high-voltage technology division with national and international responsibility for gas-insulated switching systems. In 2003 he took over the management of the Leibniz Institute for Plasma Research and Technology e.V. as Chairman and Scientific Director and was appointed professor at the University of Greifswald.
Konrad Falko Wutscher	Managing Director at SFC Umwelttechnik GmbH Konrad Falko Wutscher is a senior consultant for the process technology for physical – chemical – biological treatment of water and wastewater of any nature and origin. He has been involved in significant projects both as a consultant and a technology provider. His experience not only includes countries in Europe but many regions worldwide where water re-use and pollution control are becoming of major importance.

AFFILIATED INSTITUTIONS

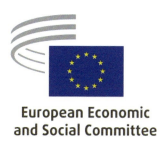

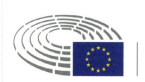

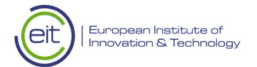

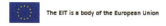

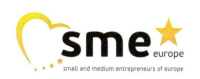

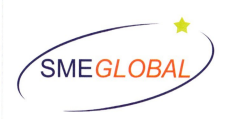

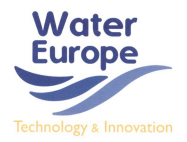

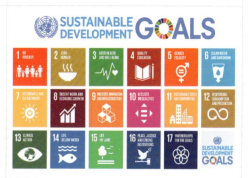